Midwives and Management

A Handbook

Rosemary E. Cross

Books for Midwives Press

B)n

Published by Books for Midwives Press, 174a Ashley Road, Hale, Cheshire, WA15 9SF, England.

© 1996, Rosemary Cross
Reprinted 1988
First edition

ISBN 1-898507-20-1

British Library Cataloguing in Publication Data
A catalogue record for this book is available from the British Library

Printed in Great Britain by Cromwell Press Ltd

Contents

Dedication and Acknowledgments

This book is dedicated to those managers and educationalists who gave me opportunities and had faith in me and to all those midwives and student midwives I had the pleasure of working alongside. It is to them I owe the inspiration for this book.

Also my grateful thanks to friend and colleague Chrisitina Tucker, for conscientiously reading the text and her sound advice, and to Catherine Bryant, Editor, and Henry Hochland, Publisher, for their unfailing belief and support.

Preface

This book is written for midwives. Midwifery managers responsible for the organization and management of Maternity Services, midwives who would like a better understanding of what management is about and students undertaking diploma and degree midwifery courses. It is an attempt to combine academic and practical and focus on issues that particularly concern midwives. The content is deliberately broad, covering topics from management and leadership theories, NHS changes and their consequences, stressors in the workplace, teamworking, providing quality services, ethical and moral issues and personal techniques for success. The content evolves from my experience in management, teaching and practice.

The idea for a book of this kind came when I was working as Director of Midwifery and Nursing Services. To do my job effectively I searched the numerous management texts and literature available to me, but frequently wished there was a book which consolidated all aspects for Maternity Services management. Of course a book this size does not presuppose to have all the answers but it will provide that focal point.

I hope the contents of this book will help towards better understanding and will encourage a corporate responsibility among midwives in management and practice. Midwives and midwifery managers are constantly in contact with people and consequently the qualities of effective communication and leadership are crucially important. If these are not developed then effective management cannot proceed. The common goal for midwives is to provide the best possible care for all mothers and babies, and it is only through shared experience this can be achieved.

The term 'Maternity Services' has been used generically and includes neonatal services and other services that contribute to the provision of a fully integrated maternity service. 'Midwifery manager' can stand alone, or be interchanged with 'midwifery sister' or 'team leader'. Reference to midwives and managers is in the feminine gender but no discrimination is implied.

Although this book is written for midwives I hope it will be of value to those in the nursing profession, general managers, medical staff and other 'interested' readers who want to know more about the Maternity Services and how it is managed.

CHAPTER ONE

The Past, The Present, The Future

*'To achieve a shift in emphasis in development policy for the Maternity
Services will require energy, determination and leadership at all levels
of the NHS – it will not come about by merely wishing.'*
(Health Committee, Second Report, Maternity Services 1991-92)

An historical perspective of midwifery

The history of midwifery and maternity care goes back to the beginning of time.
Childbirth was associated with 'Mother Earth' and considered a female 'mystery' which
only women understood. In ancient times there are references made to the work
carried out by midwives. A Mochica sculpture (c.500 BC), unmatched in the ancient
history of medicine, plainly shows a woman in parturition. Behind her sits a helper or
midwife endeavouring to ease the delivery by pressure or massage and the child's
head is being held between the hands of a second midwife who kneels down in front
of the woman in labour. Socrates, whose mother was a midwife, considered midwifery
a most respected profession, and Aristotle said the office of a midwife, being a helper
of nature, was most necessary. Further he said she must have a cheerful and pleasant
nature, and never be in a hurry, though her business may call her to some other case,
lest she should thereby endanger the mother or the child. Kitzinger (1988) tells us that
Tao Te Ching (c.500 BC), in describing the role of the midwife, said she should do
good without show and fuss, and if she must take the lead, ensure that the mother is
helped, yet still feels free and in charge. In Roman times, Soranus said midwives
should be intelligent and literate, to enable them to study theory as well as practice
their art, and some midwives of that time were skilled in medicine and surgery as well.

There are also biblical references. In Exodus i, 16–21, it is recorded that midwives
Shiprah and Puah disobeyed the King of Egypt when instructed to kill all male babies
of Hebrew women delivered by them. They feared God and saved the 'men children
alive', and God dealt well with the midwives and gave them houses. In Genesis
xxxviii, 27–29, reference is made to a midwife conducting a twin labour. It is recorded
that when the first twin put out its hand she bound upon it a scarlet thread. The baby
then withdrew its hand, and his twin brother was born first. Afterward the second twin
was born with the scarlet thread upon his hand.

In England, until the sixteenth century midwifery was practised entirely by women.
Their skills were based on knowledge and practices passed from one generation to
the next. According to Da Cruz (1967) the birthing stool was one such practice handed

down through the generations. Most midwives were middle aged married women who had themselves borne children. By the fourteenth century the Christian Church had included in their campaign against heretics the prosecution of 'witches', and thus began 'two hundred years of anti-witch mania' (Donnison, 1988). During this time thousands (mostly women) died. Despite being the 'wise women of the village' midwives throughout the dark ages were tortured and burned as witches. They practised a mixture of common sense, experience and superstition, the latter being an accepted part of medical practice at the time. It is recorded that in 1481, a Yorkshire midwife, Agnes Marshall, was prosecuted for using incantations and for lacking the necessary experience and skills for midwifery. Although the Christian Church tolerated women as healers in subservient roles it was intolerant of women who dared to practice independently, and the first formal arrangement for the control of midwives was made in 1512. Under Henry VIIIs Act to regulate physicians, women practitioners were licenced with the men.

During the sixteenth century the midwifery book, *The Birth of Mankynde*, by Eurharius Roesslin, was published in English. Although this was credited as being one of the earliest and most popular midwifery books (Beekman, 1979) it was of little use to the majority of midwives because they could not read. In the introduction of the book, comment is made on the reception the work received when first made available to midwives and reads as follows:

> 'Let not the good midwives be offended (though I have called some midwives indiscreet, unreasonable and churlish) for verily there is no science but that it hath its apes, owls, bears and asses which, as above all others have most need of information and training [yet] will kick and whine against such as would reform or reduce to any better way than they have been accustomed to times past'.

Midwives during the seventeenth century varied in competence and disposition. In his book, *Observations on Midwifery*, Percy Willughby referred to the country midwives as being 'illiterate women, of the meanest sort, who not knowing how otherwise to live, had taken midwifery up for getting a shilling or two'. Better educated midwives did exist, who had spent years working alongside an experienced midwife, often their own mother, before 'hanging out the sign of the cradle' (Donnison, 1988). In 1671, the first textbook written by an English midwife Mrs Jane Sharpe of London, was published, entitled the *Midwives Book.* She directed her book to her sisters, 'the midwives of England', and said her reasons for writing the book were because of the 'many miseries women endure in the hands of unskilled midwives'. The book contained much good sense and some superstitions, but most importantly Mrs Sharpe sensed how much midwives were threatened with the advent of men-midwives. Although men only attended difficult or abnormal births, Mrs Sharpe feared that since midwives lacked theoretical and practical knowledge, men might become more preferred than women. How right she was. Changes in the seventeenth century had a profound effect on the way midwifery was provided. Men began to practise midwifery, even though the majority of midwives opposed it, as did most of the general public. According to Kitzinger (1988), it was from this time that midwives were expected to concede to doctors, who had greater prestige by virtue of their profession and gender.

Donnison (1988) asserts there was another potent force at work during the seventeenth century that greatly influenced the future of midwives. This was the 'new philosophy' of Descartes (1596–1650) and Newton (1642–1727), that advocated rational and experimental enquiry as the highway to 'scientific truth'. Most already accepted the Aristotelian belief that rationality was a male quality, and that women were physically and intellectually inferior to men. For the new philosophy to progress thinkers had to eradicate the 'female' from their understanding and raise up a 'masculine philosophy', which would lead to the discovery of 'masculine and durable truths'. Donnison adds that the impact of the masculine mechanistic philosophy should not be underestimated. It dominated scientific thinking for nearly three centuries and still plays a central role in medical thought today.

Attempts to regulate midwifery and to gain recognition for the profession of midwifery were tried by the Chamberlen family of men-midwives. In 1616 Peter Chamberlen proposed to James I that 'some order be laid down by the State for the instruction and civil government of midwives' (Da Cruz, 1967) but this failed. A further attempt was made by Peter Chamberlen, his nephew, in 1633, but this also was not successful. However, Witz (1992) argues these attempts allegedly masterminded by the Chamberlens were intended to grant monopolies to them rather than midwives. It was a London midwife, Mrs Elizabeth Cellier, who petitioned to James II in 1687 for a Royal Charter and stressed the need to educate and regulate midwives (Donnision, 1988).

By the middle of the eighteenth century the number of men-midwives had substantially increased. Men-midwives began to achieve distinctions and respect for their work, and to gain hold on the better paid midwifery. William Smellie made detailed studies of normal labours while attending hundreds of poor women in London, and began to give practical and theoretical teaching to doctors and midwives, even though the majority of midwives were still opposed and resentful of men-midwives. Midwives were particularly opposed to Smellie because of his interest in normal childbirth. Witz (1992) remarks that moves to educate and regulate midwives were necessary because men-midwives were encroaching on a traditionally female sphere by observing the practices of midwives. From the seventeenth century men-midwives had sought to deskill the midwife by restricting her role to 'attending' and not 'intervening' during labour. Witz maintains that later medical men engaged in a demarcation strategy of deskilling which centred around the distinction between normal and abnormal labour. They sought to ossify the division of labour, whereby the medical profession could supervise, contain and control midwifery practice.

During the nineteenth century the novels of Charles Dickens attempted to draw public attention to the kind of people who were entrusted to care for the sick and to women in childbirth. The creation of the character Sairey Gamp in his book *Martin Chuzzlewit* (1844), as the poor and uneducated 'monthly nurse' illustrated the appalling low standards of midwifery that were being practised. Dickens chose not to use the word 'midwife' because of its lowly status. The incompetence of ignorant midwives also became a continuing theme in medical journals, under the title 'Midwives Midwifery' and they regularly included reports of fatalities (Donnision, 1988). Of course, good midwives did exist, and a few were to be found in villages attending the wives of small tradesmen and farmers, where records tell us they gave of their best for little reward. The better educated midwives were to be found in the cities and larger towns, and some had salaried posts in hospitals and workhouse infirmaries, or worked as 'out-door' staff of unions, hospitals or charities (Donnision, 1988). Generally, however, the situation was one of decline for midwives. Not surprisingly the middle classes began to prefer 'obstetric care' to that provided by the traditional midwives, who were left to look after the working classes and the poor. Most midwives struggled to survive themselves, frequently taking on other jobs such as washing and charring.

Despite the decline in the midwife's position, some members of the aristocracy and the middle classes resisted the emergence of men-midwives and refused to employ them. Another factor was the belief that male attendance at birth had a corrupting effect on society. Supporters of midwives continued to promote midwifery as a suitable occupation for middle class women who had to earn a living. Educated daughters of medical men and clergyman continued to enter midwifery, and the Ladies Obstetrical College was founded in London in 1864. Florence Nightingale also attempted to pioneer the efficient training of midwives, but a training scheme she organized with the Kings College Hospital London, was not a success. In 1872, the London Obstetrical Society (founded in 1858) set up its own Examination Board with its own diploma, anticipating this action would finally lead to legislation. Reactions to this were diverse. The *Lancet* and *British Medical Journal* approved, but comments in the *Medical Times* were suspicious that a move to raise the status of midwives might be to the detriment of medical practitioners (Donnison, 1988). From 1872 the General Medical Council supported state recognition of midwives.

In 1881 the Midwives Institute was set up with the objective of gaining some kind of state recognition for midwives. The condition for full membership was the possession of the Obstetrical Society's diploma in midwifery. With money raised by the Institute, this covered the expenses for drawing up various Bills. The first of these was introduced into the House of Commons in 1890 by Mr Fell Pease. Officially promoted by the Midwives Institute, the Bill was the result of discussions between themselves, their supporters and the Council of the Obstetrical Society. The Bill was blocked at its third reading. Witz (1992) states that right from the beginning the Midwives Institute accepted the narrow knowledge base and the limited sphere of competence prescribed by medical men of the Obstetrical Society. Seven more bills were introduced unsuccessfully, the last by Mr Heywood Johnstone in 1900. He introduced this again in 1902, and it passed all three stages, receiving the Royal assent on 31 July, 1902. It had taken 12 years of controversy from the medical profession before the Midwives Act was on the Statute Book. It was 50–100 years behind most Continental countries, where the initiative had been by the government. The Midwives Institute and their supporters were jubilant. Gaining professional status for midwives was an achievement for women by women, The Midwives Institute could take credit for 20 years of hard work. Furthermore Witz believes it was the Midwives Institute's compliance with the Obstetrical Society's limited definition of the midwives' sphere of competence, that preserved for midwives a degree of autonomy in the practice of midwifery. Otherwise, it is possible the Act would never have been passed, and midwives would have lost out altogether as did North American midwives who became obstetric nurses. The Midwives Institute firmly believed that parliamentary recognition of midwives would raise the status of midwifery practice to become, as recorded in 'Nursing Notes' 1888, an 'occupation for educated, refined gentlewomen' (Witz, 1992).

Following the Midwives' Act

The 1902 Midwives Act – 'to secure better training and supervision for midwives' – sanctioned the setting up of the Central Midwives Board (CMB), and prescribed its constitution. The Board was given power to formulate the rules for the regulation of training and examinations, and to maintain a Roll of certified midwives. The title of midwife was now protected. The Midwives Institute continued to examine midwives for three years until the Central Midwives Board took over in June 1905. After this time no midwife could legally practice unless she had previously enrolled or passed the CMB examinations.

However, the 1902 Act gave the medical profession much influence in midwifery affairs. Local supervision became the responsibility of Local Medical Officers of Health, and the membership of the Central Midwives Board (CMB) had a medical majority. Furthermore, midwives were the only profession that were controlled by a body (CMB) on which its members must never be more than a minority. The CMB's disciplinary powers were also more comprehensive than the regulatory bodies of other professions (Donnison, 1988). The Rules made by the CMB outlined in precise detail the midwife's duty to mother and child.

In 1921 the 'midwives' representation on the CMB was strengthened when the Midwives Institute was invited to nominate two members (Cowell and Wainwright, 1981). They joined Miss Rosalind Paget who was in her twentieth year as a member of the CMB, and ensured midwives maintained a strong voice in the Board's considerations.

Midwives continued to work mainly independently with mothers who had their babies at home. With the passing of the Maternity and Child Welfare Act (1918) local authorities began to provide a full range of child welfare services. In addition to employing certified midwives they now employed health visitors and some authorities provided maternity homes for mothers who required institutional confinement.

Towards the end of the 1920s problems associated with childbirth began to be discussed publicly. The provision of midwives was becoming a matter of national concern and in 1928 the Ministry of Health set up a Departmental Committee to enquire into the training and practice of midwives, and their conditions of employment. In 1929 a committee was set up to examine the causes of maternal mortality which was still around four per 1,000 births (Cowell and Wainwright, 1981).

The early 1930s were difficult years for midwives. The economic depression led to immense unemployment and a fall in the birthrate, which meant there was an excess of midwives. Local Authorities were short of money and some failed to pay their domiciliary midwives fees. The Minister of Health expressed concern about the high maternal death rate in the 1930 and 1932 reports (Cowell and Wainwright, 1988). These concerns incited the medical profession towards more hospital confinements and an expansion in the provision of antenatal clinics. In 1934 the CMB made a minor revision to its rules. From that time a midwife was permitted to call herself 'state certified midwife' and to put the initials 'SCM' after her name. A third change of the Midwives Act, 'The Midwives Amendment Act', came into operation in July 1936. This raised the status of midwives by providing adequate salaries and securing prospects for midwives entering into the profession. Local Authorities could employ midwives themselves, or arrange for their employment with Maternity and Child Welfare Authorities or welfare organizations.

During the war years there was a shortage of midwives. Although more midwives were being trained they chose not to practice because pay and conditions were insufficient. In 1941, the Midwives Institute became known as the College of Midwives because of its recognition and involvement with the training of midwives. The Beveridge Report indicating the future structure of national insurance and social provision was published in 1943. A year later the blueprint for a National Health Service was published in a government White Paper, but there was no mention of midwives (Cowell and Wainwright, 1981). The College of Midwives responded by saying,

> 'The aim of the new health service should keep the midwifery service by midwives as an important and independent public service...There is unfortunately no clear-cut account of the midwives' part in the service.'

The National Health Service (NHS)

In 1948 the National Health Service Act (1946) was implemented. Funded mainly from taxes it was a health service that was to be free for all at the point of consumption. The assumption behind its implementation was that as people became healthier, costs and expenditure for healthcare would equal out or decline. But from the start facilities for healthcare provision were disproportionate, with some areas of the country having modern establishments and others being poorly resourced.

Health services were divided into three parts:
* the hospital and specialist services run by 20 Regional Hospital Boards
* general medical practitioner services and dentists, opticians and pharmacists run by Executive Councils
* the community health services run by Local Authorities, which included:
  - health centres,
  - maternal and child welfare,
  - domiciliary maternity service.

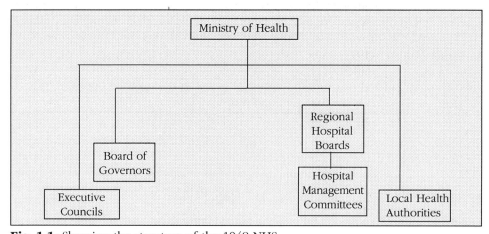

Fig. 1.1: Showing the structure of the 1948 NHS

Consequently all maternity hospitals and homes became the responsibility of Regional Hospital Boards or Boards of Governors in Teaching Hospitals, and Local Health Authorities continued to be responsible for home confinements and domiciliary midwifery practice. The Executive Councils controlled the GPs and thus the Maternity Medical Services. This meant that for the first time mothers could receive maternity services from their general practitioner without charge. Sweet (1982) remarks that this arrangement brought the midwife and doctor into closer cooperation in their complementary roles, but Cowell and Wainwright (1981) state that there was understandable apprehension among midwives as they feared they would be supplanted by the doctors. An extract from the report *Maternity in Great Britain* (1948) captures this fear by stating that 'the midwife is no mere delivery woman whose prime function is the skilful delivery of a live child. This is the climax of her task, but it started months before, early in pregnancy, and should continue at least a month after delivery'.

Each of the three parts of the NHS were separately funded and managed. According to Strong and Robinson (1992) the men and women who created the NHS believed in firm control, but the 'tight grip of ministers and civil servants unfortunately extended no further than Whitehall'. The tiers below were a different story. Ministers ruled the health service, with a workforce of nearly one million, with the thinnest of administrative veneers through delegation of power to doctors. Strong and Robinson conclude the NHS created in 1948 was brilliant but partially flawed. Brilliant because it offered real and politically viable solutions to key problems in paid healthcare. Flawed because faced with the rampant power of the medical profession, it failed for nearly 40 years to establish a proper management structure and an integrated corporate structure.

During the 1950s demands were made for extra resources and better facilities. According to Ham (1993) the 1950s were characterized aptly as the years of 'make do and mend' in the hospital service. A Ministry of Health Report (1953) on the first five years of the NHS, showed how the work of midwives was changing. This was due to an increase in antenatal clinics and an extension of attendance to the mother and baby in the postnatal period beyond 14 days. The CMB revised the Rules in 1955 requiring every midwife to attend a refresher course every five years.

The 1960s saw the creation of the Hospital Plan (1962) and several new District General Hospitals (DGHs) with modern medical facilities were built and others upgraded (Ham, 1993). Further improvements in the NHS occurred during the 1970s. The NHS Reorganization Act (1973) came into force in April 1974. The tripartite system was changed to a more unified structure, giving more attention to connecting the different parts. The reorganized structure in England (Fig. 1.2) now consisted of regions, areas and districts. Districts were based around a district general hospital (DGH) and also provided other local medical services.

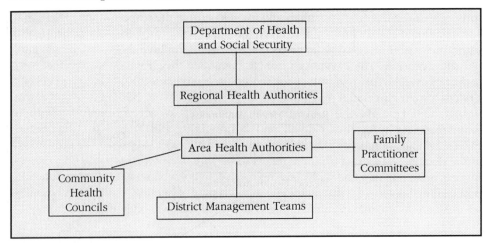

Fig. 1.2: The 1974 NHS reorganization structure

The effect of the reorganization for midwives was that it united the hospital and community Maternity Services, and an 'integrated midwifery service' was created in each district. Midwives took on more responsibilities expanding their roles into family planning, health education and neonatal paediatrics.

The Briggs Report (1972) to amalgamate the professions of nursing and midwifery had been accepted early by the government, but legislation did not occur for seven years. The main recommendation was there should be a single Central Nursing and Midwifery Council and three Boards reporting to the council for England, Scotland and Wales. The Royal College of Midwives (RCM) accepted the single Central Council on behalf of midwives, but pushed for a separate identity for the midwifery profession. Continued pressure from the RCM secured a new clause relating to the statutory Midwives Committee and protected the status of midwives. This according to Cowell and Wainwright (1981) was due to the persistent efforts of midwifery leaders. In September 1980 changes in the regulation and practice of midwives took place following the passing of the Nurses, Midwives and Health Visitors Act (1979). This saw the end of the Central Midwives Board and the beginning of the United Kingdom Central Council for Nursing, Midwifery and Health Visiting, and the creation of four National Boards for England, Wales, Scotland and Northern Ireland.

Criticisms of the reorganized (1974) NHS were swift. These mainly focused on the difficulty of establishing good relationships between the tiers and the delay in decision-making. Already it was felt there was a tier too many. Research into the new structure found it to be costly and cumbersome. The Merrison Commission (1979) endorsed one tier too many and recommended just one tier below the Region. The new Conservative government responded to the report in a consultative paper *Patients First* (1979) which proposed combining the functions of areas and districts to establish new 'District Health Authorities (DHAs)'. The result was the creation of 192 DHAs which came into operation 1 April 1982 (Fig. 1.3). Maternity Services were taken over by District Health Authorities.

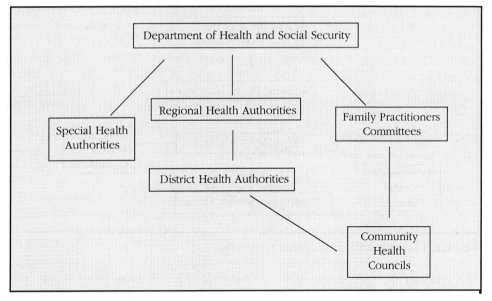

Fig. 1.3: 1982 NHS structure

The Griffiths inquiry into NHS management

Shortly after the 1982 NHS reorganization a small team, appointed by the Secretary of State for Health and Social Services and headed by Roy Griffiths, was set up to 'give advice on the effective use of management, manpower and related resources in the NHS' (Ham, 1993). The *Griffiths Report* (1983) identified the NHS lacked a clearly defined general management function and therefore there was no 'driving force' for developing, implementing and monitoring management plans. The Inquiry team stated action was badly needed for a more central strengthened NHS. It recommended general managers should be appointed at every level, and that doctors must accept the responsibility that goes with clinical freedom and be more involved in management. The government endorsed the report's recommendations and general managers were appointed at regional, district and unit levels throughout 1985 and 1986. The new general manager took responsibility for the management of the whole organization and managed everyone. According to Strong and Robinson (1992), general management was deliberately anti-professional. Specialists were essential, but to general managers 'their very virtues – if left unchecked – entailed major organizational vices'.

At local level the impact varied and general managers had freedom to create their own management structures. Very few midwives and nurses were appointed to general manager posts. The DHSS Management Board introduced performance related pay for general managers and their senior colleagues, and gave instructions on 'management budgeting' which was to be the forerunner to resource management. Lists of initiative and priorities from the DHSS kept general managers preoccupied with achieving these targets and keeping in budget (Ham, 1993). The Resource Management Initiative signalled a further change in the management of resources, as doctors, midwives, nurses and other professional staff were won over to clinical management during 1986-87.

Throughout the 1980s according to Ham (1993) a 'widening gap emerged between the money provided by the government for the NHS and the funding needed to meet increasing demand'. A review on the future of the NHS was set up in 1988, which involved a committee of senior ministers, chaired by the Prime Minister, and supported by civil servants and political advisers. During the review the DHSS, one of the largest government departments, was split into two becoming the Department of Health and the Department of Social Security. The White Paper *Working for Patients* (1989) while endorsing the basic principles on which the NHS was founded announced there was to be changes in the way healthcare was delivered. The changes would create conditions for competition between hospitals and other service providers, and to achieve competition responsibilities for purchasing and providing services were to be separated. In addition, other changes in the White Paper aimed to strengthen the management arrangements. At the Department of Health there were to be changes, with the Supervisory Board and Management Board being replaced by a Policy Board and Management Executive Board respectively. At local level Health Authorities were to be more businesslike.

Working for Patients (1989) included recommendations that would affect primary care and the community services, but it was mainly concerned with hospital services. Plans for the future of community care were contained in a response the government made to a report prepared by Sir Roy Griffiths in 1988. The White Paper *Caring for People* (1989) endorsed the Griffiths recommendations that Local Authorities were to take lead responsibility, in association with NHS Authorities, for planning community care. These changes would be in line with the new funding arrangements for care in the community.

The 'new' National Health Service

With *Working for Patients* on the statute book, new Regional Health Authorities (RHAs) were appointed. During their first meetings in July 1990 the non-executive members of District Health Authorities (DHAs) and Family Health Service Authorities (FHSAs) were appointed. The new DHAs and FHSAs had their first meetings in September 1990. Their functions were:

- to assess their residents health needs
- to plan provision for their care
- to write contracts to secure that provision
- to purchase services on their behalf.

Other early initiatives were the moves to establish NHS Trust status for hospitals and health services providers and GP Fundholding for purchasing practices. In December 1990 the government announced the first wave of NHS Trusts were to commence in April 1991. Out of 66 applications, 57 had been approved and over 100 more hospital and services had expressed an interest to be approved in the second wave (Ham, 1993). The function of NHS Trusts was to provide and manage services for which they were responsible. Some 300 GP practices were granted approval to become Fundholders in April 1991, and their function was to purchase elective services for their patients. Figure 1.4 shows the new NHS management structure in 1993.

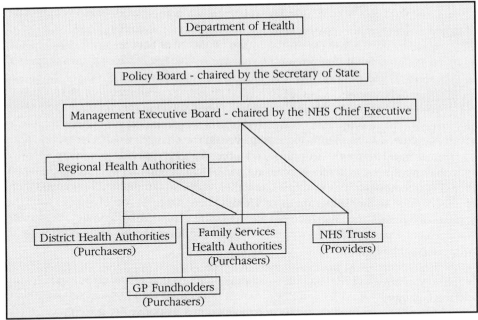

Fig. 1.4: Showing the new NHS management structure

The NHS Management Executive (NHSME)

Although accountable to the NHS Policy Board the NHSME works directly with NHS Authorities and NHS Trusts. Their functions are:

- to set objectives for the NHS in line with overall ministerial priorities and within available resources
- to monitor performance
- to provide leadership to NHS management
- to advise ministers and the Policy Board on the operation and management of the NHS.

NHS Trusts

The creation of NHS Trusts was to improve efficiency and effectiveness in the National Health Service. By establishing NHS Trusts and giving power and responsibility to those who provide the services, it was assumed the quality of care would be improved. Additionally, providers of healthcare would have to successfully compete with other providers for contracts with healthcare purchasers for them to be successful and to survive. Such a competitive environment contended the government would ensure NHS Trusts operate successful businesses and respond by putting local needs first.

CHARACTERISTICS OF NHS TRUSTS
- Self-governing units within the National Health Service.
- Run by Boards of Directors with an equal number of executive and non-executive members, who are equal in status.

- The directors have a corporate responsibility for the work done in their name.
- The NHS Trust is accountable to the Secretary of State for Health.
- The Chairperson is appointed by the Secretary of State.
- The main function of the directors is to manage the services for which they are responsible.

Freedoms include being able to:

- determine their own management structure
- employ their own staff and set own terms and conditions of service
- acquire, own and sell their own assets
- retain surpluses
- borrow money subject to annual limits.

THE FUNCTION OF NHS TRUSTS

- The Chairperson works closely with the Chief Executive in guiding the business.
- Day-to-day responsibility rests with the Chief Executive and senior executive directors.
- The executive directors on the NHS Trust Board will participate in making decisions they have to implement, and will play an active part in determining strategies and setting priorities.
- At an early stage the NHS Trust will establish a 'vision' for their services and will provide an explicit statement of the philosophy and values that guide the work of the Trust.
- Operational strategies will be developed for achieving long-term objectives.
- Strategies for monitoring will be developed to assess the achievement of short- and long-term objectives.

KEY POWERS TO NHS TRUSTS:

- to provide health services through contracts
- to run the hospital(s) or other NHS facilities vested in the Trust
- to employ staff in such numbers and on such terms as the Trust decides
- to determine pay and conditions
- to provide education and training for NHS staff
- to provide catering, domestic and recreational services for patients and staff
- to make contracts, including contracts with staff and contracts for services
- to acquire, lease and dispose of land and property required for its business
- to generate income under the terms of the Health and Medicines Act 1988
- to accept gifts, on trust or otherwise
- to borrow money, subject to the annual external financing limit set up by the Secretary of State
- to undertake joint activities with other NHS Trusts, Health Authorities etc., provided these are activities the Trust has power to undertake.

Giving NHS Trusts powers does not mean they are completely free, because each has to:

- prepare an annual business plan outlining its proposals for service delivery and capital investments
- prepare and publish an annual report and accounts
- hold an annual 'open meeting' to the public at which the annual report and accounts are discussed.

The internal market

The most outstanding characteristic about the new reforms is the purchaser–provider split, because it is an attempt of the government to delegate decision-making down to the level where health services are provided. Previous reorganizations had always concentrated on the centre – the Department of Health – insisting on accountability upwards. *Working for Patients* (1989) had the objective of facilitating and providing better quality and greater choice of service for patients. Its intention was to create a market in which providers of healthcare compete with one another to win contracts from District Health Authorities and GP Fundholders (Fig. 1.5).

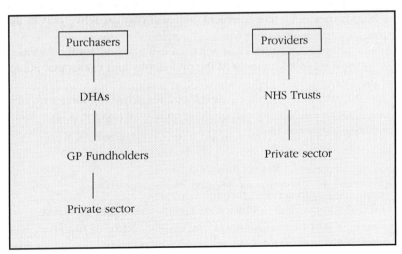

Fig. 1.5: The internal market

Purchasing organizations

DHAs have responsibility for:
- obtaining and purchasing healthcare for their local residents
- purchasing health services as either 'core' or 'non-core specialities'
- commissioning both hospital and community services.

(Core = maternity services, accident and emergency, medical; care of the elderly; Non-core = elective surgery and treatments which may involve waiting lists.)

In theory elective work can be contracted to healthcare providers inside and outside the DHA geographical area, and inside and outside the NHS. Non-residents of a district can be treated individually on an 'extra-contractual referral' (ECR) basis, which is paid for by the DHA where the person resides.

GP Fundholders have responsibility for purchasing elective 'non-core' services on behalf of their registered patients.

Private sector purchasers and providers

These tend to be focused around specific types of elective surgery, for example:
* gynaecology, in vitro fertilization (IVF)
* termination of pregnancy (TOP)
* plastic surgery
* orthopaedics.

Since the internal market reforms the use of private NHS beds and private hospitals has risen because:

* NHS purchasers contract with private hospitals to reduce waiting lists
* private hospitals contract for private beds in NHS Hospitals for elective procedures which require post-operative intensive care.

Hence contracts enable purchasers to increase their control over the amount and quality of healthcare they purchase. Healthcare providers agree to supply healthcare in accordance with the contracts agreed between themselves and the purchasers. It is envisaged competition will encourage providers to develop 'quality and value for money' services. The NHS is now a world of the internal market with:

* an increasing emphasis on consumerism
* an emphasis on value for money and income generation
* entrepreneuralism.

NHS Trusts have become 'qualities' in the market place, but 'managed competition' as it is referred to in most NHS documents, is a market like no other in the way it operates and the arguments it continues to arouse. Le Grand (Thomson, 1993) describes the NHS internal market as a 'quasi market'. He maintains that instead of an equal balance between the consumers (patients) and providers, consumers are represented by agents (purchasers) and competition.

The theme running through the NHS reforms is better management at all levels and this constitutes a major challenge to every manager. First, to recognize the NHS as a business of healthcare and secondly that business principles and methods are to be used. The emphasis is on meeting the needs of consumers, through effectiveness and quality, which is absorbed in the business plan. Marketing services and gaining the competitive edge will secure contracts and the NHS Trust's future.

However, a report by Newchurch and Co. *The Fourth Newchurch Guide to NHS Trusts Birmingham - NAHAT* (1994) says Trusts will be forced to raise money by letting or selling premises, or by merging to cut costs. The report concludes by saying 'our research suggests that more mergers are being driven from a largely financial imperative'. Mergers inevitably will not be in the best interests of local people, because they are financially driven and not clinically led.

Already there have been mergers and other types of joint purchasing agreements between DHAs. The new larger 'Purchasing Institutions' - formed by merging each District Health Authority with the Family Health Service Authority - will certainly concentrate on more specific and refined contractual agreements with providers. Kerin (1994) suggests they will be the 'champion of the people' as they concentrate on developing the health of their local population. They will continue to have strong links with Social Services, Environmental Health and Housing.

The midwife in the 1970-80s

The *Peel Report* (1970) had a profound effect on the way maternity care was provided in the United Kingdom over the next two decades. Its recommendation 'that adequate facilities for hospital confinement should be available for all women who wish it' was accepted. The trend towards 100 per cent hospital confinement was supported by the government and professionals on the grounds of greater safety of childbirth for the mother and baby. This secured the obstetric model of childbirth - that 'no birth was normal except in retrospect'. There had already been a trend towards more hospital births, from 15 per cent in 1920, 35 per cent in 1938, to 75 per cent in 1966 so it was not surprising that the propositions were readily accepted by midwives and mothers themselves. The emphasis was on safety and the message was that hospitals were better able to deal with emergencies because they had the right facilities. Therefore, it followed that home births were unsafe, as it was not possible to provide emergency facilities in the home. Further, a delay in getting a mother and baby to hospital in an emergency could cause them serious harm. Consultant obstetrician Baron (1979) wrote that 'whatever the advantages are of having a baby at home, it is not the place for an obstetric emergency'. Although midwives still believed in the normality of childbirth they were influenced by the only measure of a safe birth for mother and baby being after it had occurred. The *Short Report* (1979-80) reiterated 100 per cent hospital confinement and went even further by recommending that home confinements should be phased out altogether.

Technical procedures to make birth safer in hospital were developed rapidly. Mothers were fitted up to machines to monitor fetal wellbeing, and mechanical monitoring was used almost routinely for 'normal labours'. This was despite an early randomized study (Kelso et al, 1977) which concluded there were 'no beneficial or deleterious effects of continuous fetal heart monitoring in labour'. Labours became regularly induced or augmented, with mothers often requiring intravenous infusions and instrumental deliveries, and babies needing assisted resuscitation. A highly technical system of childbirth became the norm. The midwife became a member of the hospital team, a technician and no longer a practitioner of normal midwifery. By defining 'no birth as normal except in retrospect' this effectively took away the midwife's role, and placed all childbirth under medical control. Professor Beard speaking at the International Congress for Midwives in the early 1980s said modern technology must become a part of routine midwifery practice otherwise 'midwives will be excluded from the management of normal labour'. Kitzinger (1988) asserts that doctors became anxious about their role and intervened in perfectly normal labours because the technology was waiting to be used and they had been trained to intervene. The emotional aspect of caring for mothers in labour took on a completely new meaning as midwives strived to provide the vital elements of care in an impersonal clinical environment.

Concerns about the care of mothers and babies, and the midwife's role were not only restricted to the hospital. Research carried out by Robinson, Golden and Bradley (Robinson, 1989) showed that many women were having routine antenatal examinations twice, because doctors repeated the procedure after the midwife. Not only was this inconvenient to the mother, it was a waste of resources and an insult to the midwife because it implied her clinical judgement was inadequate. In the postnatal period doctors duplicated midwives work, and midwives had to obtain doctor authority prior to transferring a mother and baby home. At the time O'Brien (1981) commented 'midwifery as an art is disappearing now childbirth has become part of the "health industry", a hospital occasion presided over by obstetrical entrepreneurs, usually male, in conditions of depersonalised asepsis which transforms women'.

General practitioner (GP) unit confinements began to replace births in the home, but a strict booking criteria meant only mothers who had a previous successful pregnancy and delivery were suitable. Primigravidae mothers were excluded. The DOMINO scheme - domiciliary midwife in and out - became quite popular, with mothers being transferred by the midwife into the GP unit during early labour, and the mother returning home with her new baby within 48 hours of birth. A minority of mothers still requested home confinement, but usually the mother was pressurized to change her mind by emphasizing the danger to her unborn child, and more than often she agreed to give birth in the GP unit.

Childbirth became a great media interest. Views were expressed in newspapers and womens journals, and on radio and television. Mothers were worried that technical procedures to make birth safe were making them less important than the machines. Hill and Taylor (1977) of the Association for the Improvement in Maternity Services wrote 'the mother's presence often appears to be ignored as scientists battle to control her womb and its function, using weapons such as the electrocardiograph to monitor the fetal heart'. An article on how to enjoy having a baby in the 'Woman' magazine (Horwood, 1979) told mothers how to demand their rights when entering Maternity Hospitals. Toynbee (1986) writing in the 'Guardian' newspaper criticized the 'natural childbirth' lobby and said mothers were still 'proper women' if they chose the reassurance of fetal monitors and an epidural for a pain free labour. The conclusion that women should be able to choose for themselves became paramount. Commentators were also concerned about the future of midwives, as they saw their role being eroded by obstetricians.

Discussions to agree practice and legislation for the Euromidwife took place during the 1970s but agreement was difficult because of the diverse ways midwives practised across the continent. In May 1977 no agreement had been reached for the length of training, but still the CMB issued a revised syllabus to increase the training to eighteen months. The government agreed in principal but no money was available. In early 1980 the CMB issued a further midwifery training syllabus, this time with financial backing. The main objectives for extending the training were to provide more in-depth theory and to allow more time for clinical experience Additionally there had been concerns that immediately following the one year training only half the midwives practised, the other half returning to general nursing or to another branch of nursing. It was envisaged the new eighteen month course would encourage more midwives to stay in the profession.

If midwives roles were being eroded, what about midwifery managers? More than often midwifery management was the responsibility of a Principal Nursing Officer (Midwifery), with Senior Midwifery Officers each having management responsibility for the hospital services, community services and midwifery education respectively. However, in some Districts nurses began to take over the management of midwifery, with Divisional Nursing Officers having responsibility for the integrated Maternity Services and Midwifery Schools. A prerequisite was usually a midwifery qualification, but this was not essential. Criticisms about midwifery management emerged during the late 1980s as midwives questioned the rigidity of local midwifery policies and what they considered 'the bureaucratic style of managers'.

Throughout the 1980s mothers and midwives challenged the interventionalist process of birth. Increasingly midwives carried out research and began to dispute the accepted obstetric procedures. Sleep et al (1984) in their perineal trial of two thousand women said they could find little support for liberal use of episiotomy. In 1987 Flint and Poulengeris published their *Know Your Midwife* report advocating the benefits of continuity of midwifery care and recommending the implementation of team midwifery. Systems of individualized care developed to give mothers more choice, and schemes to make Maternity units less clinical. In 1987 the first planned underwater birth in the country took place in Royal Leamington Spa, with midwives working closely with the mother to achieve her request. The trend that followed involved midwifery managers, midwives and mothers throughout the country setting up 'waterbirth' services, often with opposition from general managers and doctors. Mothers and maternity-consumer organizations continued to vocalize their dissatisfaction about the impersonal care mothers received and the lack of choice and control they had during pregnancy and childbirth. Articles, such as 'My Baby wasn't born, she was torn from me' continued to make the headlines in 1990. Tew (Walton and Hamilton, 1995) challenged the safety of hospital births versus home births, by showing statistically a correlation could not be made between a fall in perinatal mortality and hospital confinements.

'Changing Childbirth'

Towards the end of the 1980s, mothers and midwives had become very articulate about the type of maternity care they wanted, which was a return to a more natural style of childbirth. Most importantly mothers said they wanted to have more say in decisions surrounding their birth and maternity care. The Association of Radical Midwives published their proposals for mothers to be central to care in *The Vision* (1986), which also emphasized the importance of continuity and better use of midwives skills. The Royal College of Midwives endorsed women must be full partners in care in their publication *Towards a Healthy Nation* (1987). A House of Commons Health Committee was set up in 1992 to look at the future of Maternity Services, and took evidence from individuals, professional and consumer organizations and government departments. The Health Committee Report (1992-93) had much to criticize on the way maternity care was provided, but particularly the current policy to encourage all women to give birth in hospital. It concluded that 'a medical model of care should no longer drive the service and that women should be given unbiased information and an opportunity for choice in the type of maternity care they received, including the option, previously largely denied to them, of having their babies at home, or in small maternity units'. The Health Committee Report was greeted with enthusiasm by mothers and midwives. In response to the Report the government set up an 'Expert Committee' to review NHS policy for maternity care and to make recommendations.

In March 1993 invited speakers - professionals and users of maternity services, an invited panel and the 'Expert Committee' plus representatives from each Health District, education institutions and professional and voluntary organizations gathered together for a consensus conference organized by the Kings Fund for the Department of Health. The lively debate echoed many concerns about the way Maternity Services were provided and suggestions were put forward for more women-centred care. Although there was acknowledgement that tensions existed between the professions it was agreed there was no place for professional rivalries. A written statement was drawn up following the conference, and sent to the 'Expert Committee' as evidence and for their consideration.

Now the scene was set for changes that would reform the way maternity care was to be provided in this country. In some strange way midwives were in the strongest position they had been this century. The Report of the Expert Maternity Group *Changing Childbirth* (1993) with its theme of 'women centred care, control, choice and continuity', was published in the autumn. After a three month consultation period the government announced the recommendations were to be implemented in full. Midwives were now on the threshold of putting into practice one of the most revolutionary childbirth reports there has ever been.

Three key principles of good maternity care are stated:

- The woman must be the focus of maternity care. She should be able to feel that she is in control of what is happening to her and able to make decisions about her care, based on her needs, having discussed matters fully with the professionals involved.
- Maternity Services must be readily and easily accessible to all. They should be sensitive to the needs of the local population and based primarily in the community.
- Women should be involved in the monitoring and planning of Maternity Services to ensure that they are responsive to the needs of a changing society. In addition care should be effective and resources used efficiently.

Implicit in these three statements is the shift required for the future provision of maternity care. The report is divided into five chapters, with objectives and action points to be met by the purchasers and providers of Maternity Services. Indicators of success to be achieved within five years are as follows:

1.   All women should be entitled to carry their own notes.

2.   Every woman should know one midwife who ensures continuity of her midwifery care - the named midwife.

3.   At least 30 per cent of women should have the midwife as the lead professional.

4.   Every woman should know the lead professional who has a key role in the planning and provision of her care.

5.   At least 75 per cent of women should know the person who cares for them during their delivery.

6.   Midwives should have direct access to some beds in all maternity units.

7.   At least 30 per cent of women delivered in a maternity unit should be admitted under the management of a midwife.

8.   The total number of antenatal visits for women with uncomplicated pregnancies should have been reviewed in the light of available evidence and the Royal College of Obstetricians and Gynaecologists guidelines.

9.   All front line ambulances should have a paramedic able to support the midwife who needs to transfer a woman to hospital in an emergency.

10   All women should have access to information about the services available in their locality.

Emphasis on the role the midwife is to play in maternity care is explicit. Purchasers and providers are asked to ensure midwives make full use of their knowledge and skills by developing schemes that reflect the full role for which they have been trained.

Implementing the *Changing Childbirth* recommendations will require midwifery managers and midwives to work closely together. Discussing the report and its purpose, and working through each of the objectives will provide an opportunity for a review of services to be carried out. This will help to establish a strong sense of alignment between the purpose of the Maternity Services and how to reach the desired results. This will enable a new philosophy for maternity care to be decided. Of course to meet the needs of local mothers and the purchasers of Maternity Services strategies for change would have to planned and agreed.

It also means midwives and midwifery managers identifying training needs. Managers obtaining resources for training and development and supporting midwives in the changes. Many midwives working today were trained and practised through the era of technology, and many will require retraining and help in adjusting to a more autonomous practitioner role. It is a time for midwives to come together and help each other and not to be divided. Midwives and midwifery managers must grasp opportunities for innovation within the boundaries of the report and take a lead in a way they have not done before. Innovation is about making changes. An innovative midwife - whether a practitioner or manager - is one who takes the lead, has a vision and believes in what she strives for in advocating the best care for mothers and babies. Innovators like leaders have to be risk takers - risking failure as well as success and accepting at the onset that explanation and energy will be required. Midwifery managers must drive these changes, and midwives must have confidence and work with their managers. Professor Lesley Page (Read, 1994) says it is now up to managers to support midwives as they implement the changes, but it also up to midwives to support their managers in reorganizing the way maternity care is provided and the way midwives work. Walton and Hamilton (1995) maintain that if midwives do not meet the challenges and grasp the opportunities they could become mere obstetric nurses. Kelsall (1993) in her analysis says 'it is not education or training, but changes in attitude that midwives need if they are to be able to give their clients choice, continuity of care and consumer-led maternity services.'

Some Maternity Services will be well advanced with implementing the recommendations, others will be in the early stages. As Piercy and Downe (1995) remind us moving to a women-centred system of care requires a fundamental change in the organization of care, particularly in the organization of midwifery services. They believe to achieve the kind of service specified by *Changing Childbirth* it is clear that providers must agree with purchasers a mechanism for evaluating and monitoring progress. Purchasers and providers need to look not only at the effectiveness of interventions, but at their cost-effectiveness so as to maximise health gain for their population. Purchasers should have drawn up their strategic plans during 1994/95 with initial targets for change being introduced during 1995/96.

Jackson (1995) says it is extremely important that concerns about *Changing Childbirth* are voiced and explored. This is an essential part of organizational change, and midwifery managers must establish with midwives the strength of their feelings about the recommendations, and any anxieties and needs they may have. Jackson affirms *Changing Childbirth* stresses the necessity for Maternity Services to be responsive to changing needs and to research evidence, and this philosophy should equally apply to the implementation of the recommendations.

What of the future?

Changing Childbirth aims to put women and their families at the centre of maternity services, by giving mothers choice, continuity and control. To achieve these goals mothers, midwives, doctors, other professionals, managers and consumer groups will have to work closely together. In this sense opportunities for midwives have never been greater, because they can put ideas forward, be innovative in their practice and take a lead in planning the future of maternity care.

The challenges for midwives are boundless, and midwives must decide what they want professionally and where they want to be in the future. Midwifery is a dynamic profession and boundaries will expand and change over time. Midwifery diploma and degree courses prepare midwives to be critical, reflective and creative practitioners, and able to practice in any setting. Perhaps now is the time to radically review and challenge some of the long-held clinical practices and organizational arrangements such as those described below.

NHS practice or independent midwifery practice

'Midwife-Led Units' in NHS hospitals can provide comfortable environments where mothers have choice and immediate access to other facilities if necessary. Do midwives want to run and develop these? Also with more NHS Trusts 'subcontracting' services the possibility of 'buying in' chunks of midwifery services for groups of mothers is not so remote. Does this open up more opportunities for 'practices' of independent midwives being bought into the NHS for the provision of maternity care.

Team midwifery

There are various possibilities for different models of teams to be developed. For example, the 'Nuffield Model', based on a small case load for midwives, supports the benefits for continuity of the carer. It is envisaged most teams will operate in the community, but what about using the maternity unit as a focus for team midwifery? Utilizing the enormous amount of midwifery expertise already there. Small midwifery teams could function in the maternity unit and also go out to mothers and babies in the community (Fig. 1.6).

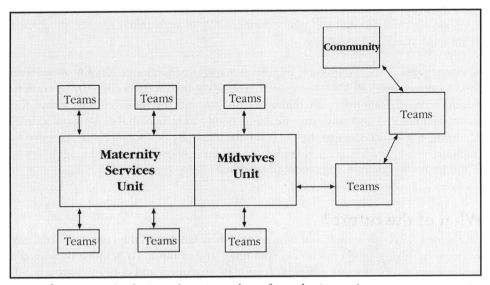

Fig. 1.6: Team Midwifery working in and out from the 'centre'

Specialization in midwifery

Is now the time for two types of midwifery practitioner? The specialist of 'normal' midwifery with skills to undertake a full range of practice throughout pregnancy, labour and postnatally and the specialist of 'high dependency' midwifery practice, who works in the labour suite and the hospital setting? Supporters of creating two specialist models argue that too much is being expected of midwives today, by requiring them to practice the full range of clinical skills and to be proficient in so many situations and settings. By separating 'high dependency' midwifery, practitioners who choose to specialize would extend their knowledge and skills to be accountable for advanced clinical practices e.g. setting up intravenous infusions, forceps deliveries and first assistant for caesarean sections.

Complementary therapies

Should midwives expand their role into acupuncture, homeopathy, herbalism, aromatherapy and spiritual healing? Already a number of midwives practice acupuncture for mothers in pregnancy and after birth. The National Association of Health Authorities and Trusts in their research paper *Complementary Therapies in the NHS* (1994) said there was a growing public demand for alternative therapies and a growing professional interest. Although mothers are fortunate to receive high quality maternity care, many are increasingly searching for alternative therapies to enhance the healthy functioning of their body.

Supervision of midwives

Would one full time clinical Supervisor of Midwives in each NHS Trust be more efficient and effective than the present supervisory arrangement? The current system has two main flaws - role conflict between the managerial and supervisory role and lack of available time for Supervisors to execute their role effectively. Also clinical midwives appointed as Supervisors of Midwives often experience difficulties with their peer group, whom they have to supervise. Another question is - do midwives need Supervisors? Some midwives believe that their professional accountability removes the need for a Supervisor of Midwives.

Towards the twenty first century

The publication of the Department of Health discussion document *The Challenge for Nursing and Midwifery in the 21st Century* (1994) indicates there are great changes ahead for nursing and midwifery. It says that at best the professions can win enhanced status, at worst they can be broken up and marginalized. Nurses and midwives are warned by the United Kingdoms' four Chief Nursing Officers that 'to sit and wait for the future to surprise us carries the risk of confusion and waste'. Therefore, midwives must challenge traditional boundaries and decide what they want to do, where and when.

Summary

A historical perspective of midwifery

The history of midwifery can be traced to ancient times. In England during the fourteenth century, the Christian Church in its campaign to drive out heretics tortured and burned midwives accused of witchcraft. The midwives struggle to gain recognition can be traced to 1512 when the first formal arrangement for control was made. The advent of men-midwives affected midwives grievously during the seventeenth and eighteenth centuries. Men-midwives gained prestige and recognition for their work, whilst midwives remained unskilled and lacked theoretical and practical knowledge. The midwives position further declined during the nineteenth century when they were relegated to attend the poor, whilst doctors attended the upper and middle classes.

Efforts to gain midwifery state registration lasted more than twenty years, culminating in the *Midwives Act* (1902). This led to the setting up of the Central Midwives Board to regulate training and examinations, and maintain a roll of certified midwives. From this time until the commencement of the National Health Service (1948) midwives worked mostly in the community, independently or with Local Authorities.

The National Health Service (NHS)

The history of the NHS, from its inception and through the 1974 and 1982 reorganizations, reveals the difficulties of implementing a 'brilliant policy' on such a large scale. From the start health care facilities were inequable, funding for hospitals, GPs and community services were separately managed, the medical profession dominated and decision-making was delayed. The *Griffiths Inquiry* (1983) identified the NHS lacked a clearly defined management structure which led to the appointment of general managers at regional, district and unit levels during 1985-86. Griffiths also stated that doctors should have stronger involvement in management and during 1986-87 the Resource Management Iniative saw the beginning of clinicians in management. Throughout the 1980s funding required for health care exceeded that provided by the government. This led to *Working for Patients* (1989) which announced changes in the way health services were to be delivered, and the creation of the purchaser and provider split.

The new NHS

NHS Trusts (providers), District Health Authorities (main purchasers) and GP Fundholders (purchasers) have been set up and given responsibilities, powers and accountability for ensuring users of their health services get the best care. The new health service is now the world of the internal market, one in which providers compete with one another to win contracts from purchasers. The emphasis is on consumerism. The intention is that competition will encourage providers to develop quality services that are value for money.

The midwife in the 1970s and 1980s

The *Peel Report* (1970) had a profound effect on the way maternity care was provided. The move towards 100 per cent hospital confinement enforced the obstetric model of 'no birth is normal except in retrospect'. Technical procedures became the norm. The midwife's role was eroded. Mothers and consumer groups expressed dissatisfaction about routine procedures and their lack of control. Midwives carried out research and challenged accepted obstetric policy. Childbirth became a public concern, with views being aired in the media. Midwifery publications *The Vision* (1986) and *Towards a Healthy Nation* (1987) stressed women should be central to their maternity care.

'Changing Childbirth'

The government's Health Committee Report 1992-93 had much to criticize with the way maternity services were being provided, and stated the 'medical model' should no longer drive maternity care. The subsequent report *Changing Childbirth* (1993) with its theme of 'women centred care, control, choice and continuity' sets out principles and objectives for purchasers and providers to achieve, and indicators for success. Implementing *Changing Childbirth* will require midwives and midwifery managers to work together with doctors, mothers and consumer organizations. Many midwives will need support to re-establish their practitioner role. Opportunities have never been greater - the future is in the hands of midwives. Challenges are boundless, and midwives must decide where they want to be now and in the future.

CHAPTER TWO

Management and Leadership

*'Every managerial act must be seen an unequivocal support for
urgency in pursuit of constant testing, change and improvement.'*
(Tom Peters, 1988)

What does a manager do?

The meaning of management to the majority of people is mostly misunderstood. Despite numerous and varied definitions, and attempts through observation and research to make it a more academic and professional discipline, still the meaning of management eludes most people and has emotive connotations. Ask managers what they do and often they have difficulty in telling us. This is not surprising because a manager's job is full and varied. Ask subordinates what managers do, and although the majority have little idea the very question can unleash strong emotions about 'the management'. A strange thing has happened. Inadvertently, in their response, there has been a change to the term 'management' and yet the question relates to the manager. Somewhere, the manager as a person has become lost, and replaced by the neutral and abstract word of 'management'.

That organizations change over time is not in doubt and according to Handy (1993) we are constantly being reminded that times change increasingly faster. During the last five years radical changes in the way the National Health Service is managed has seen the rise of NHS Trust Chief Executives being given power within the Griffiths (1983) General Management Structure. Yet at the same time management within Trusts has become 'flattened'. What in reality is happening, is that as NHS Trusts take over the management of local services, there has been a demise of the 'middle manager', and more responsibility has been devolved to the clinical level. Gone is the hierarchical management structure, which most midwives and nurses are used to, and in its place has come the flattened structure where more responsibility is given to staff holding senior clinical, ward and departmental positions.

What does this mean for midwives? Realistically it means that those holding a management position take on a bigger span of control, with more staff reporting directly to them. The advantages for midwives working in such a structure, as Andrews (1994) points out, is that it gives them more opportunity for local autonomy and decision-making. Now it is not necessary for midwives to go right to the top of the organization, because decisions can be made and implemented at a lower level.

However, for local midwifery managers this means that as they take on more management control, simultaneously there will be an increase in the number of midwives reporting to them. This means more inter-personal relationships have to be made. To stay on top of the job, a wide range of skills and techniques are required. Not just for survival, as too much energy can be lost in 'hanging on', but for enjoyment, success and fulfilment in all that they do.

The process of management is important to midwifery managers, and to midwives who seek to affect the behaviour of others. Midwifery managers work for NHS Trusts and carry responsibilities for achieving the Maternity Services goals, but managing is much more than this. It is about leadership, teamworking and communicating, and motivating staff to provide a Maternity Service they can be proud of, through meeting the needs of mothers and babies.

The management process

A simple definition for a manager is 'someone who gets things done through the activities of others', but management is a highly complex process. Based on the traditional approach management may include all or any of the following.

Forecasting, planning and development

This includes looking ahead to the future, planning and developing the Maternity Services through setting objectives, implementing arrangements and systems and continuously looking ahead to improve the service of the future. Planning requires foresight and vision. It includes identifying problems and agreeing short and long range goals.

Managing human resources

'The people factor' – directing, managing, delegating, educating, training and developing midwives and support staff within the corporate strategy and the culture of the Maternity Services and the NHS Trust. It involves taking the planned Human Resources strategy and 'bringing it alive'.

Policy making

Agreeing goals and targets through consultation and setting objectives for Maternity Services provision. A policy being an internal guide to be followed to achieve the Maternity Services objectives.

Organizing

Providing the resources – primary (human) and secondary (non-human, e.g. money, equipment, buildings, time) – and bringing them together to fulfil the Maternity Services goals and provide a service which is effective, productive and safe.

Communicating

Guiding, influencing, talking to, talking with, listening to, sharing with and understanding individuals and groups of individuals within the Maternity Services, the NHS Trust and externally. This includes communicating with staff (subordinates and colleagues), senior managers, the customers of the Maternity Services – mothers and purchasers, and external groups e.g. National Childbirth Trust, Community Health Council and the media.

Motivating

Developing a willingness in others to be directed which is achieved through leadership, delegation and empowerment. Motivating midwives and support staff is an important factor in determining how well they perform and the level of quality they achieve in their practice and the work they do.

Coordinating

Pulling together and harmonizing the responsibilities and activities of others for achieving successful outcomes in maternity care, for individual midwives and support staff and the overall success of Maternity Services.

Controlling

Making sure things happen the way they are planned and evaluating progress and outcomes. If necessary it includes adapting and changing, as differences and deviations can occur with plans, targets, budgets and the way staff perform. Controlling includes clinical reviews, quality audit, consumer satisfaction surveys and feedback, and monitoring Maternity Services statistics. Successes are recognized, rewarded and celebrated.

Information handling

Receiving, reading, disseminating, sharing, and storing reports, relevant documents and special information, for the benefit of the Maternity Services, self and other individuals, e.g. midwives, medical colleagues, mothers. It also involves transmitting information to the NHS Trust Board, purchasers of maternity care, and to 'outsiders' about the Maternity Services, including plans, policies, actions and results

Problem solving and decision-making

Identifying problems, gathering and sharing information and deciding plans of action (with others) to solve problems, initiate improvements and bring about change to shape the future Maternity Services. It includes representing Maternity Services for important organizational negotiations, dealing with disturbances and implementing corrective action.

Effective skills in each of these responsibilities is a requirement for the midwifery manager to do the job successfully. There is, however, a common theme running throughout each of the above components, and this is the power and importance of communication.

As far back as 1967, a major British research project involving a large 'sample' of managers and supervised by Stewart (Handy, 1983) found that managers spent on average two-thirds of their working time in conversation of one type or another. This is a useful reminder of the significance of communication, but at the same time, as Boot et al (1982) remind us 'management is not a neat and tidy unitary concept but rather a general term in need of continual redefinition according to time and circumstance'.

Management theories

There are some distinctions between management and leadership theories, although in reality the difference is less clear. Management and leadership is intrinsically linked, and some knowledge of management theories will help midwifery managers understand why managers and workers function in particular ways, and behave the way they do.

Scientific theories

These early theories explored how to achieve the maximum rate (the limit) from each worker. They focused on 'workers in factories, and those employed in assembly lines', and centred on how to increase productivity, by concentrating on the time it took a person to do a task(s). As a result, the selection of employees was based on factors associated with activity and appropriate training, so as to achieve high productivity. These formed the basis of time and motion studies.

The Human Relations School of management theory

This theory was developed in the late 1930s and 1940s and focused on the weakness of the scientific theories, in that analysis of the task alone was not sufficient. Through research a number of factors were identified that had an immense impact on productivity. These included the attitudes of the workers, any personal problems they might have and how much support they received to do the job.

Motivational theories

These theories maintain the principle that the effective manager-leader is the one who will increase productivity through creating an environment that is supportive for each individual worker by encouraging satisfaction and removing factors that will restrain and hinder. In 1960 and 1966, McGregor (Benton, 1994; La Monica, 1994) postulated that all humans can be seen in one of two ways:

1.   Theory X - the average person:
        - is lazy
        - not too intelligent
        - lacks motivation

- finds work distasteful
- is reluctant to take responsibility

McGregor asserted that people had these traits because the organization or past experience made them that way.

2.   Theory Y - is in contrast to the assumptions of Theory X
        - work is natural when the conditions are favourable
        - the average person is self directed
        - is motivated according to needs
        - is self-controlled if properly motivated
        - can solve problems

McGregor concludes that manager-leaders can provide opportunities and the right atmosphere where work will be motivating and fulfilling by:

- removing obstacles, problems and difficulties
- providing guidance and encouragement
- identifying skilful and talented people so that optimum performance can be achieved.

In 1966, Herzberg (Benton, 1994) developed Theory Y by identifying the 'needs' that affect a person's motivation to work. These he divided into two groups:

- needs adjusted to avoid discomfort, insecurity and pain, such as appropriate salary, safe and healthy work environment, good interpersonal relationships and education and training.
- needs required for emotional growth: include delegated responsibility, job satisfaction and advancement opportunities.

Situation theory

This theory contends that the scientific and motivational theories have left out a major factor - the environment.

In 1971, House (Benton, 1994) developed the 'Path Goal Theory' based on the assumption that a person's motivation to perform a task is related to:

- achieving a desired outcome
- personal satisfaction
- reward

Therefore, the manager's role in Situation theory is to:

- assess the person's competence
- estimate the probability of success
- anticipate any problems and obstacles
- provide support
- give appropriate reward

Management skills

According to La Monica (1994) there are three general categories of skills that managers must possess:

- technical skills
- human skills
- conceptual skills.

These were first classified in 1955 by Katz and adapted to the field of behavioural sciences by Hersey and Blanchard in 1988 (La Monica, 1994).

Technical skills

The ability to use relevant knowledge, methods, techniques and equipment for the performance of specific practices, assignments and tasks acquired through experience, education and training.

Human skills

Ability and judgement when working with and through people, which includes an understanding of motivation and the use of effective leadership.

Conceptual skills

The ability to understand the complexities of the overall organization, and where one's own role and responsibilities fit in. This knowledge enables the manager to perform according to the goals of the total organization rather than just the goals of their own section or group.

Research has shown that managers, according to their level and position in the organization, will require different levels of technical and conceptual skills to perform their responsibilities effectively. Human skills remain constant at all levels, taking up the greater part of the management function.

An acceptance that the balance of skills will vary according to a manager's position in the organization should help midwives to appreciate the differences in role function. For example, the midwifery manager, in addition to requiring human skills, will need a balance of technical (practical) and conceptual (wider theoretical) skills, whereas the midwifery sister will require extended technical skills and less conceptual skills.

Figure 2.1 shows the balance of skills that are required by the midwifery manager and midwifery sister, compared with the NHS Trust Director of Nursing and Midwifery.

Efficient managers will rely on a number of management skills, techniques and methods, and not any single approach. The effective midwifery manager will be the one who can achieve a balance between the requirements of the Maternity Services, the needs of the staff and herself. When direction, leadership and support are given to staff in a clear and educative way this will facilitate them to achieve their goals, and for the overall success of the Maternity Services.

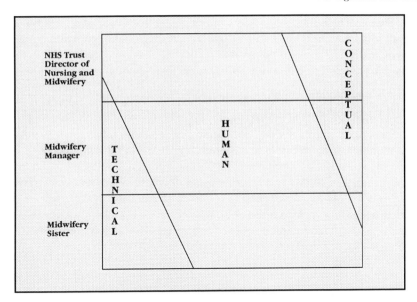

Fig. 2.1: Showing management skills according to level of management

Leadership

Leadership and management are intertwined. Although there have been attempts by management theorists to separate the two, the purpose and function of management cannot be separated from that of leadership (see below).

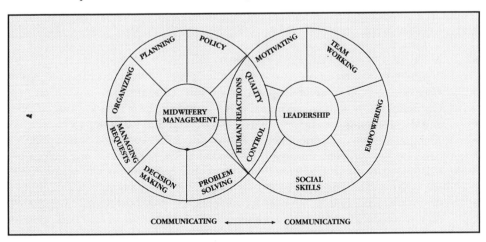

Fig. 2.2: Showing the overlap between management and leadership

Numerous definitions of leadership exist but they all converge on two main points:

- leadership involves using communication processes
- leadership influences the activities of others towards attaining goals.

In 1973, Fleishman (La Monica, 1994) pointed out that leadership always involves attempts to influence, and further more that all interpersonal relationships can involve elements of leadership. This is important to midwives, as this recognizes that in providing maternity care, midwives can influence mothers as leaders.

Midwifery managers, as well as having skills in planning, organizing, budgeting, decision-making, will also need to have well developed leadership skills. As Wall (1989) wisely states 'the manager, in establishing the legitimacy to manage, has to be worthy of that position, demonstrating not only knowledge but a skill in handling others'.

Leadership is not an exercise of authority, using power to obtain personal prestige and reward. Nor is it a matter of stepping out in front and hoping the rest will follow. The true leader, according to Margaret Schurr (1968), does not claim power by virtue of position but realizes that status is earned, and that allegiance comes when she has gained the confidence and respect of those for whom she is responsible.

Qualities of leadership

The fact that a midwife is exceptionally skilled in her professional practice does not necessarily make her a natural leader. Whilst it is true that midwifery managers can be trained and educated in management skills, they must first possess the basic qualities from which leadership skills can be developed. These are the fundamental values of human behaviour, the foundation on which all human relationships depend.

Basic qualities

* Understanding: an ability and readiness to accept that 'people' react differently to situations and have diverse needs.
* Ability to seek cooperation: being able to plan and work with others towards a common goal, based on mutual respect, welcoming ideas and contributions of everyone to achieve an atmosphere of tolerance and respect.
* Communication skills: an acceptance that communication is a two-way process, and that listening is as necessary as it is to talk and to be understood.
* Ability to delegate: a confidence to entrust and empower others. An inability to delegate will prevent successful leadership - not only will a non-delegating manager become overwhelmed and incapable of performing her own work, she will deprive others of the chance to find fulfilment in theirs.
* Wisdom: an ability to make wise judgements and decisions is vital. Acceptance by a manager that she cannot know all the answers but knows how to seek help and accepts this willingly and courteously.

Personal qualities

A leader is a person whose own character is one of harmony. Someone who possesses, through self-knowledge, an appreciation of the needs of others, and through a balanced, impartial approach can control and direct a situation, and at the same time bring out the best in others.

- Values and beliefs: the special personality of the individual will influence the quality of leadership.

- Integrity: essential for all those who are in anyway responsible for others. A 'natural sincerity' and consistency means others will know they can trust that person and will not be let down. It is usually the integrity of the manager and not her position which will command respect

- Moral courage and tenacity: when others see moral courage in action, they take note. Staff will recognize the determination which guides and controls a leader in various situations, and will appreciate the person who stands by them through difficult times.

- Self control and self respect: someone who has learnt to understand herself is in a position to exert control over others. A manager who has the ability to accept that she has weaknesses and is sufficiently modest to acknowledge and do something about them possesses 'poise', which in turn produces self respect.

- Sense of humour: leadership should be enjoyed - any contact with people has the potential for happiness. A cheerful appearance and an element of encouragement and enjoyment must come through if others are to feel their contribution is valued.

Theories on leaders

Trait theories

Trait theories are the earliest theories, developed in an attempt to understand leadership behaviour. They are based on leaders having innate qualities and characteristics, suggesting that 'a leader is born and not made'.

Characteristics such as:
- above average intelligence
- strong sense of 'self'
- highly motivated, energetic
- courageous
- persistent, ruthless
- above or below average height
- good health.

By identifying these traits it was supposed that leaders could at least be selected, even if they could not be made. However, as Handy (1993) reminds us, trait theories rest on the assumption that the individual is more important than the situation. This in itself is a major flaw, especially as leadership concerns the involvement of others, the job to be done and the circumstances.

Two further criticisms of the trait theories are:
- possession of all or some of the characteristics does not guarantee effective leadership
- possession of all of the traits is almost an impossible ideal.

Behavioural functional theories

Theories based on leader-behaviour styles submit 'it is not who the leader is that is important, but what the leader does '. There are three typical classifications for leader behaviour - autocratic, democratic and laissez-faire.

AUTOCRATIC

- often described as authoritarian
- a firm leader who makes unilateral decisions
- usually gives orders to be obeyed without question
- communication is from 'top-down'.

DEMOCRATIC

- often described as participative
- a leader who becomes part of the team
- involves the group in decision-making
- communication is 'top-down', 'bottom-up' and 'side-side'.

LAISSEZ-FAIRE

- often seen as 'doing nothing'
- maintains only loose control over the group
- recognized as 'leader' only because of formal position in the organization
- considers staff can lead themselves.

By plotting these leadership styles, from autocratic to abdication (Fig. 2.3) it can be seen that as the leader moves more towards participating and becoming part of the team, this correspondingly gives staff more responsibility and power.

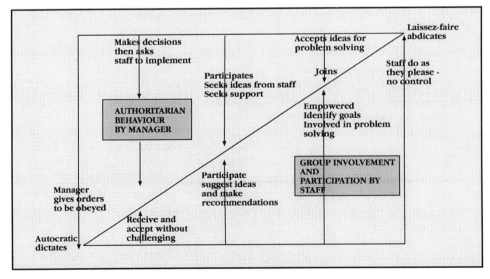

Fig. 2.3: Leadership styles from autocratic to abdication

Informal surveys on the opinions of 'leaders and followers' according to La Monica (1994) usually result in the democratic style of leadership getting the most votes. But she adds that although the 'beauty of the democratic style is the participants choice, this is not always appropriate'. In reality a manager needs to use a mixture of leadership styles at different times, but the skill is in knowing which one to use and when.

Situation leadership theory

More recent studies have suggested that leaders are better described in terms of their orientation towards both tasks or relationships. Although all leaders exhibit these tendencies to some extent, by using 'leadership models' they can be characterized as being high or low to tasks and relationships.

The situational leadership theory model (Fig. 2.4) as developed by Hersey and Blanchard in 1988 (La Monica, 1994) contains the two components of task and relationships along separate axes. By completing the four quadrants with high or low to tasks and relationships this will give four leader behaviour styles, which can be interpreted as follows:

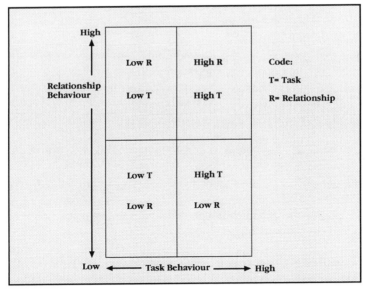

Fig. 2.4: Four leader-behaviour styles

HIGH RELATIONSHIPS AND HIGH TASKS
* make the best leaders
* balances the desire to get the task completed with concern for the needs of the staff-group
* uses open communication and involves the team actively in agreeing and setting goals
* the leader is still in full control although the staff-group are participative

HIGH TASKS AND LOW RELATIONSHIPS

- directive and controlling approach
- the leader defines the task, explains it to the staff-group and tells them when it is to be done
- communication is one way and the staff-group is expected to do as they are told

HIGH RELATIONSHIPS AND LOW TASKS

- the leader's first concern is for the staff-group, how to get them together to complete the task
- although the leader might identify the problem for the group there is little planning and the staff-group are left to work things out for themselves

LOW RELATIONSHIPS AND LOW TASKS

- the leader keeps a low profile, although may be contacted by the staff group for consultation
- by delegating to the staff-group the leader shifts the control to them

Contingency theories

These suggest that good leadership is conditional, and what makes a good leader is more dependent on the people and the situation. Blake and Lawrence (1989) contend that contingency theories take into account behaviour dimensions of the task, people and their participation, and Handy (1993) also includes the leader's position within the specific staff-group. The three behaviour dimensions of Blake and Lawrence are:

- task centredness - the extent to which the task is taken seriously and rationally pursued
- people centredness - the extent to which people are valued, motivated and cared for
- participation - the extent to which colleagues and staff-groups are involved in plans and decision-making.

Blake and Lawrence suggest that if contingency theory is crossed with the above behaviour dimensions, three practical leadership propositions will emerge.

TASK CENTRED LEADERSHIP

- suitable for staff carrying out naturally unstructured tasks.
- tends to raise the level of staff performance and enhances job satisfaction.
- not suitable where tasks are highly structured, with little room for manoeuvre and repetitive.

PEOPLE CENTRED LEADERSHIP
- supportive leadership.
- tends to be effective for tasks and situations that are stressful, uncertain or frustrating.
- by supporting staff this underlines their own contribution and its importance, raises self-confidence and positively influences morale.

PARTICIPATIVE LEADERSHIP
- keeps staff well informed.
- involves staff-groups in planning and decision-making processes and gets them more committed to achieving agreed goals.
- gives staff more control over their work which is generally good for morale.

Transforming leadership

'We hear a great deal nowadays about the crisis of leadership. In fact, the phenomenon is nothing of the sort. It is a crisis of "followship".' (Francis Kinsman, 1986)

With the move towards the use of more information technology in Maternity Services and the shift away from the hierarchical management system, a new type of leadership is needed to deal with these changes. Today's midwives and support service staff want to participate and be at the forefront of decisions concerning the provision of maternity care. Hence tomorrow's midwives will demand different kinds of practice-agreements based on changing skills, and the new style leader will not only require a tactful whilst motivating manner but also a flair with people. Kinsman (1986) further believes that tomorrow's leader must be regarded as the 'first among equals', and that their major attribute will be to empower colleagues to be their own leaders.

Ritscher (1986) on the other hand believes that one of the basic functions of tomorrows leadership is to stimulate and focus the organization's spirit. He is not using the word spirit in a religious way, but claims the spirit of an organization is its heart. Spirit is a sense of vitality, energy, vision and purpose. All organizations have spirit, but in some cases it is dull and tarnished, and if managers and leaders do not meet the challenge of enspiriting an organization, it will be blown to the prevailing winds. Only an organization that is well grounded in its spiritual nature has the will and the strength to survive.

This type of leadership is very much in tune with today's maternity services. Midwifery managers and midwives may feel compelled to create different styles of leadership to bring about the changes required for *Changing Childbirth* (1993) and at the same time provide a Maternity Service that is focused and in harmony with providing high quality care in a climate of balancing resources and competition.

Ten qualities of spiritual (transformational) leadership

(Adapted from James A. Ritscher, 1986)

These qualities are inner and spiritual. They do not involve 'doing' as much as 'being'. If you have the 'being' worked out, the 'doing' will come naturally. The reverse is not true.

1. Inspired vision - Leadership involves creating a vision that draws people forward towards a common-desired reality. The cohesive force is spiritual rather than mechanical.

2. Clarity of mind - This is the core of leadership, to be able to create ideas that just come almost effortlessly. This is the submerged portion of the 'iceberg', the solid foundation out of which the active portion of leadership springs. For clarity of mind it is necessary to plan 'non-doing times' during the day, for meditation and clear thought processes.

3. Will, toughness and intention - Leadership is transcendental. It is a bold existential act of courage and will. When you assume a position of leadership you move away from the pack. Toughness is not opposed to openness and sensitivity.

4. Low ego, high results - Strength is different from ego. Strength is vital for a leader to push forward and achieve results. Ego is over-emphasis on self. Inflation of ego is at the expense of others. The antitheses of ego is caring, service, dedication and excellence in one's work.

5. No separation - This is something of a paradox. Because there is a strong tendency of others to experience a leader as separate, transformational leaders have learnt how to reduce this sense of separation. In other words, the 'others' know the leader is inherently separate but they experience a sense of intimacy and connection - charisma.

6. Trust and openness - This helps to create integration and cohesion in the workplace. Trust is having faith in others and self. Openness is being unguarded, candid and truthful. A leader brings tough-minded optimism to a situation. Trust creates a powerful energy around a leader.

7. Insight into human nature - This is a skill of human interaction. Leaders are characterized by their ability to read, interpret and guide the actions of others. It is a connecting force that touches people at a very deep level. It is impossible to 'touch this level' if you have not reached this level yourself.

8. Skill in creating people structures: groundedness - A transformational leader knows how people function in groups, and understands group dynamics. They have exceptional skills in facilitating groups to maintain 'group focus'. They believe groups can be trustworthy and that organizations can work. They create open trustworthy meetings.

9. Integrity - This creates an experience of soundness, robustness and vigour. An organization without integrity is 'limp and invites worms and parasites'. An

organization with integrity is strong, like a well-rooted tree. Each person in the organization has a tendency to do that which is praiseworthy, effective and right. The person who has the most to do with establishing this quality is the leader. The leader must talk about integrity and practice it.

10.   A context of personal growth and fulfilment - A transformational leader is a person who catalyses a dedicated close-knit organization that pursues a common vision and produces effective results. People working in such an organization have a deep respect for themselves and each other. They bring 'something of themselves' to work. People feel ready to take on challenges. They are ready to fulfil the vision.

Personal qualities and skills necessary for success

Achieving success will benefit the organization and at the same time give personal satisfaction and raise self-esteem. There are proven techniques and skills to enhance achievements that have been tested and used by effective managers which will make all the difference between success and failure.

At first glance many of these techniques appear basic and self-evident, but by following these skills midwifery managers will be able increase their ability to do their job well, will create more energy for themselves and will be helped to appreciate the contribution of colleagues

Image: confidence and assertiveness

Confidence breeds confidence in others. A midwifery manager who is assertive instils confidence in those around her and at the same time colleagues will begin to recognize and enjoy these qualities in others. Two-way communications will be enhanced and colleagues will feel trust and respect for the manager.

- Create a good image. Dress well, feel good and get noticed.
- Walk a bit faster than average and with a purpose. Keep your eyes to the front and do not look down.
- Smile frequently and meaningfully.
- Volunteer for jobs, projects and committees that will bring you in contact with other people in the organization, as well as your own staff.
- Work for quality and always do your best. Be reliable and become someone your boss, colleagues and subordinates can rely on.
- Give off an aura of confidence and more people will believe in you. You will attract admiration and people will seek you out.
- Create an achieving style – remember first impressions only come once!

Getting the job done

Have a strategy for success. A midwifery manager's job is demanding and techniques of self-motivation are required. A single-minded approach is essential otherwise personal goals will not be achieved and your staff will not be motivated to reach theirs.

- Think positively and focus on your goals.
- Have your goals written down. Keep them written down and easily accessible. Display them, don't file them or hide them away.
- Set deadlines and keep to them.
- Select and work on the important, not what suddenly appears urgent.
- Keep in perspective what is important and work towards results. Do not work for work's sake and become bogged down.
- Treat the inevitable difficulties as a challenge and convert problems into opportunities.
- Take time to relax and time to think.
- Face difficulties and fears and write them down. Do not avoid difficult tasks. Look at ways of tackling them and keep to your plan.
- Have outside interests and keep healthy.

Managing effectively

Effective managers are those with good communication skills. To manage successfully requires confidence and sound interpersonal skills. Dealing and forming positive relationships with people is essential to get work done and reach desirable outcomes for the organization and yourself.

- Never take orders without discussion. Always question and challenge them.
- Be honest with your boss. Keep your boss up-to-date and tell her or him what is going on, even if the news is not good.
- When in discussion with your boss, present your own views and when you have alternative, constructive proposals let them be known.
- Accept responsibility for your 'sphere of midwifery management', and for mistakes and errors of judgement within your department.
- Get on with your job and 'do things without constantly checking back'. If you are not sure what to do or how to do it, seek advice and clarification.
- Ensure your subordinates understand clearly what their jobs entail and what their responsibilities are. Give them a written job description but ensure it is accurate and up-to-date.
- Praise your subordinates when they do well and give them credit for achievements. Take corrective action for unproductive behaviour and when things go wrong.
- Help your staff develop their capabilities and potential, through appraisal and staff development reviews. Help them to identify and develop their training needs and motivate themselves.
- Delegate work to your staff. Try not to do everything yourself. Delegation gives subordinates experience in management skills and can enhance personal satisfaction and commitment.
- Pursue and defend the Maternity Services interests but do not do this to the exclusion of the interests of the NHS Trust.

The eyes have it

Facial expression is crucial to communication, but must correspond with the words we speak. It is no good praising someone with a frozen smile on your lips or making calming statements with a scowl on your face.

Eye contact can be very powerful. If you want to get noticed use your eyes to your advantage. O'Brien (1992) reminds us that eye contact should be clear and intermittent. Direct staring, on the other hand, can be intimidating and a 'put-you-down' for the other person.

- Let your eyes express the message you wish to convey.
- If you want to observe and find out more about a person sit further away. Sitting too close to someone face-to-face will cause them to look down, turn away or narrow their eyes.
- The more eye contact you have with a group of people the more likely you are to be accepted as their leader.
- Scientific studies have shown that if a group of people with no designated leader is seated around a table, the leader usually emerges from the side of the table with fewer people, because they will have more visual contact with more people.
- When chairing or leading a meeting sit in a position where you can oversee the group.
- It is harder to start an argument with someone sitting side by side as eye contact is reduced.
- Remember a person being encouraged to say negative or embarrassing things will avoid all eye contact.

Personal efficiency

Self-management is frequently neglected, but to achieve ultimate success a number of basic techniques will improve how your office is organized. Your secretary is your most valid ally, and once you have agreed key ways to handle your mail, the telephone and your diary, you will have more time to spend on essential management responsibilities.

Ask your secretary to sort the incoming mail into:

- urgent action
- for circulation to the team, wards or departments
- reply and response
- information only
- scrap and stop unwanted mail.

Plan each day at the onset, or better still the day before.

- Set secretary times.
- List times for jobs and phone calls.
- Ask your secretary to follow these up.

- Set times to see staff either in your office or in the clinical areas.
- Develop a routine.
- Develop a diary-planning format.
- Let your secretary organize your diary.
- Adopt a diary system which will allow for detailed timings and also sections for undertaking routine tasks, correspondence and telephone calls.
- Have two diaries - one for yourself and one for your secretary - but let your secretary have yours each day for updating and amending as necessary.
- Programme small blocks of time for thinking and reflection. Let people know when you do not wish to be disturbed.
- Be ruthless with the telephone (Pearson and Thomas, 1991) and use it to your advantage to get results.
- Plan a time each day for outgoing phone calls.
- Use your secretary to get the list of people you want.
- Have a policy of not taking incoming calls - operate a 'call-back' system.
- Ask your secretary to screen callers and to record the time of the call, name of the caller and a brief message.
- Ask your secretary to handle routine calls, and if necessary reroute to another person in the team.
- Devise a central filing system and give your secretary responsibility for this. Ensure you know how the filing works as you may need reports and papers urgently. Don't let filing pile up - it is better to do it yourself than to let important documents get lost in a mound of paper.

Handling, reading and disseminating written information

The amount of paper coming into your office can be overwhelming. We are told by Treacy (1991) that millions of working hours are wasted in processing paperwork which should never have been introduced in the first place. Dealing promptly and effectively with incoming paperwork will pay off, give you more time, keep your desk clear and result in lower stress levels.

- Deal with each item of paper as soon as possible after it arrives on your desk or in your in-tray.
- Keep your in-tray off your desk so that it doesn't distract you.
- Handle each piece of paper only once. Don't pick it up and leave to be dealt with later – this will only have to be dealt with twice.
- Be selective in your reading or you will become 'crushed' beneath the load. Scan long reports by reading the contents page or headings, the summary, conclusion and recommendations. Look for charts, figures, graphs etc.
- Decide what to do with each item of paperwork
  - act on it
  - pass it on to someone else to read/summarize or act on
  - file it
  - throw it away
- Ask your secretary to highlight sections as above.

- Prioritize your paperwork to act on:
  - high priority: anything which directly benefits or effects your department of 'sphere of management', i.e. complaints, revenue costs, budget returns, waiting times, untoward incidents, sickness and absenteeism.
  - deadlines to be met and reports to be completed by an agreed date.
  - information promised to staff, other departments, purchasers.
- Ensure midwives and anyone in your team include a front page summary when sending you reports or proposals.
- Keep your desk clear. Start and end your day with a clear desk. Cluttered desks lead to distraction, lost papers, delay in decision-making and procrastination. Time is then spent on catching up on yesterdays paperwork instead of planning for tomorrow

Summary

A simple definition for a manager is someone who gets things done through the activities of others, and yet the meaning of management is mostly misunderstood. This is not surprising because management is not a unitary concept but a highly complex process.

Changes in the configuration of NHS Trusts have favoured a move away from the hierarchical management structure to one that is flattened. This means more management responsibility and control has been given to clinical midwifery managers and midwifery sisters, and a wide range of knowledge, skills and techniques are required.

By breaking down the traditional management process into ten components, different roles and responsibilities can be identified. Communication is a theme which runs through each component, emphasizing the importance and power of effective communication in management. Knowledge of management theories facilitate an understanding of why managers and workers behave and function in the way they do. To perform effectively managers require technical, human and conceptual skills, but the balance of technical and conceptual skills will vary according to the manager's level and position in the organization. Human skills remain constant at all levels, taking up most of the manager's time.

Effective managers are also effective leaders. Management and leadership are intertwined. Although there are some distinctions between management and leadership theories, in reality the difference is less clear. Managers can be taught management skills, but for the growth of leadership managers must first possess basic personal qualities and a belief in the fundamental values of human behaviour. Transforming leadership is about empowering others to be their own leaders. This can be achieved through focusing on the 'spirit' of the organization - its vitality, energy and vision. Spiritual leadership does not involve doing as much as being. By considering, the ten qualities of spiritual leadership, midwifery managers may wish to develop these for leading tomorrows midwives.

Established skills and techniques are an asset to any manager, not only for personal achievement but to accomplish success for the organization. Many of these techniques may appear basic and self evident but by using them, managers can create more energy for themselves, perform more effectively and gain the respect of others. Assertiveness, self-motivation, forming positive relationships, eye contact, personal efficiency and dealing with paperwork are some of the techniques worth cultivating.

CHAPTER THREE

Problem Solving and Decision-Making

'Decision-making is like moving from darkness to light. A problem is solved, only for it to reappear and submerge us into darkness again'
(Helga Drummond, 1991)

Effective decision-making is about formulating events, bringing about results and shaping the future. Whereas making a decision is 'to cut' or 'to determine a course of action', the decision-making process involves events leading up to a chosen moment and beyond.

Moreover Drummond (1991) believes that as well as action, the future can also be shaped by 'inaction' or decisive-inaction, which stems from so called 'non-decision making', and this can deliberately thwart change (Fig. 3.1).

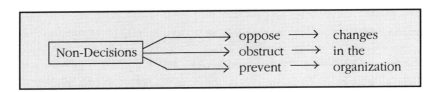

Fig. 3.1: Showing the effect of decisive 'inaction' on the organizations

Further more, a so called 'decisionless-decision', which is usually a small unplanned decision, fails to consider the long term implications of a change, and usually results in 'entrapment'. Entrapment results in the decision-maker making more and more short-term decisions to overcome the decisions that have gone wrong. In other words, the decision-maker continues despite obstacles, persisting and refusing to accept defeat (Fig. 3.2).

Escalation in decision-making

(Adapted from Helga Drummond, 1991)

1. Initially decisions are taken in small steps, often in a reactive or unplanned way. This is known as 'incrementalism' and deals mainly with problems in the short-term.

2. Escalation occurs when the decision-maker becomes 'trapped in their loosing-course of action' due to their previous incremental decisions. The choice is to withdraw or persist. Quitting can be expensive in economic and/or personal terms.

3. Once in the trap the decision-maker may persist because:
   - persistence makes the decision-maker/manager look like a leader whatever the reality
   - failure is punishable thus the temptation to hide it by 'escalating'
   - persistence is a way of signalling to others that 'you are right'
   - maintaining appearances can be disastrous in decision-making.

4. Feelings of disappointment raise escalation. Escalation is higher when a decision-maker is responsible for the original decision.

5. Competition stimulates escalation. Once competition starts, escalation grows and intensifies. Competition becomes destructive if the desire for revenge becomes dominant.

6. The only way to get out of the escalation-trap is for the decision-maker to accept and admit there is a problem, and acknowledge the decision was the wrong one.

7. To prevent escalation occurring again the decision-maker must carry out a full evaluation of their decision-making processes. The use of structured 'economic and scientific' models will go some way in preventing escalation and entrapment in the future.

Fig. 3.2: Showing how 'Entrapment' can manifest

Types of decision-making

There are three main types of decision-making as far as Maternity Services management is concerned:

- Strategic decision-making
- Operational decision-making
- Personal-Professional decision-making

Strategic decision-making

Strategic decision-making is concerned with organizational policy and direction, forward planning, business planning, how the Maternity Service functions and operates, and where it is going in the future. Strategic decisions, therefore, have implications on whether the Maternity Services will grow and on its future survival.

Operational decision-making

Operational decision-making is concerned with day-to-day management of the Maternity Services - in the wards, clinics and the community. Decisions made at this level are crucially important, because strategy depends on successful and effective decision-making at the level where care is actually provided - at the 'sharp-end'.

Personal-Professional decision-making

Personal-Professional decisions are those made by midwives, and are concerned with standards of professional practice, working towards raising the quality of maternity care and teamworking. Personal decisions on their own usually only effect the person involved, but when combined with professional standards and teamworking, they will have beneficial effects on the service as a whole.

Of course, the opposite is true. If a decision is made by a midwife not to participate in setting standards and not to work as a team member, this would adversely affect the quality of care provided and lead to a breakdown in inter-personal relationships.

Management decision theory

This derives from the economists of the early industrial era and proceeds from the assumption that decision-makers are motivated to maximize profit or potential benefits (Drummond, 1991). The logic of this is - 'that if the decision-maker can maximize profit this is preferable to an average profit'. For example, although a decision-maker would be content with £50.00 profit, all things being equal a £100.00 profit would be preferable.

This concept is known as utility or maximization, but the key to decision-making in any organization is dependent upon rationality of the decision-maker.

Rationality in this context means acting in a manner consistent with maximizing gain. It applies to all decision-making in the management of the Maternity Services, and not just for managing budgets. For example, providing midwives with in-service training to update their professional practice would also raise the standards of care for mothers and babies. This in turn would contribute to the Maternity Services achieving the agreed contract standards with the purchasers, which could lead to a larger contract with them in the future.

Morgan (Handy, 1993) considers decision-makers should function like 'machines' because it is only then that they can become insusceptible to emotion and to outside influences. Of course this is unrealistic, but it is worth remembering that however objective a midwifery manager may consider herself, being human in itself creates a susceptibility to outside influences and the manipulation of others. Drummond (1991) says decision-makers 'require a sense of their own vulnerability'. Although it is virtually impossible to prevent others from trying to influence the decision-process for their own ends, with insight at least this should reduce the liability to manipulation.

The traditional approach to decision-making

The Synoptic Model

Although many versions and variations of the Synoptic Model exist, it generally involves the following sequence of steps:

1. Recognize and identify the problem - by giving yourself special planned time for identifying opportunities for decision-making.

2. Define the problem - by referring to the causes - past and present - rather than the symptoms. For example, for high staff sickness first the reasons of sickness must be identified before you can begin to look at ways to improve the situation.

3. Clarify and prioritize goals - by reassessing the objectives of the NHS Trust and the Maternity Services, and looking ahead to the future.

4. Generate and consider options - by 'brainstorming' you should be able to come up with a range of alternatives on how to solve the problem. This can be done on your own or with a group of staff who share the problem.

5. Evaluate options - by considering each option in detail, and what effects each alternative option would have on the Maternity Service and the NHS Trust.

6. Choose a solution and implement - by choosing the solution that most maximizes gain and is consistent with the goals you have set for the Maternity Services.

   Once you have chosen the solution, you must make sure that the staff who will be responsible for carrying out the decision:
   - understand why it has been chosen
   - know how to implement the change
   - actually carry it out.

7. Evaluate the decision - by monitoring the implementation is successful. This will enable you to assess whether the solution can be further improved.

What this Synoptic Model provides is a framework within which you can work. It has a prescriptive approach which should facilitate rational decision-making. Its value is in its simplification and its progressional-logical sequence. Decision-making is an art and a science (Drummond, 1991). Therefore it is important to be systematic and logical.

Failure to use such a model, or one of the 'scientific models' could mean you simply use intuition. Making intuitive decisions according to Sutherland (1992) causes a person to become irrational. However, recent justification for the use of intuition in strategic planning has been made by Hadridge (1995), who maintains managers should acknowledge the value to be gained from intuition and creativity as well as analysis.

Unfortunately the Synoptic Model is not as easy to use as it may at first appear. This is not because the model is inappropriate, but because decision-making itself is involved and complicated. However, it is still essential to use a model, not only because of the risk of total intuition, but because without a framework it is difficult to deal with the vast number of issues surrounding even the most simple of problems.

Some difficulties with decision-making

Difficulties with problems

- Decision-making begins with a problem, but in reality problems do not suddenly appear.
- Often the midwifery manager or the organization may not even be aware that a problem exists because the staff keep it to themselves, and when a problem is identified this may not be correctly defined.
- Problems are often ignored until they become a crisis.

Difficulty with determining problems

- A possible definition for a problem could be an abnormality or departure from the 'norm', due to some cause which needs a solution to resolve it.
- To be able to recognize and then define a problem depends on having the correct information. This is often not easy to obtain and sometimes crucial data may even be unobtainable. Frequently information about a problem is restricted to gossip and rumour, and staff may be reluctant to give details to managers.
- Information-gathering is only part of attempting to determine the problem. Being able to interpret the information is critical, but if the information is incomplete mistakes in decision-making can be made.
- It cannot always be taken for granted that a problem is always understood. Sometimes those that make decisions are unable to grasp the problem, and occasionally they are not even interested in solving it.

Difficulties with clarifying and prioritizing goals

Assuming a problem has been correctly diagnosed, the next stage is to prioritize the goals or the objectives. Goals are the 'future states' which the Maternity Services is striving to reach i.e. for quality, growth and survival. Unfortunately in practice, managers when carrying out decision-making often operate without goals, or without really understanding what the goals of the organization mean and how they can be achieved.

Difficulties with decision-making that is timely

Decision-making is often delayed because the necessary information is not forwarded on time. Also because managers frequently experience 'work-overload' due to insufficient delegation (Handy, 1993), this can further compound the delay.

An effective method for obtaining information in decision-making

A good plan is to treat the gathering of information as a fundamental part of the decision-making process.

1.   First work out for yourself:
        - what information you require
        - how you want the information to be presented and given to you
        - the way you are going to communicate your requirements to others.

2.   Talk to the staff about the issue, this will also help you breakdown the problem more clearly. Additionally this will assist you to identify which staff will be able to help you.

3.   Initially information-needs are more associated with understanding the problem. This phase is important if you are to fully comprehend what is happening and the significance of the problem.

4.   Write summaries of key points, and use 'flow charts'. These are useful for facilitating understanding and clarifying the problem.

5.   As you obtain early information you will need to review your information needs. Any previous requests which you now decide will be 'surplus' to your requirements should be cancelled immediately. It is far better to do this than waste other peoples' time and energy in providing information you do not want.

6.   Once you begin to understand the issues surrounding the problem, you will be able to see what other definite information you require. When asking questions or requesting more information be specific, and give the exact details of what you want and how you want it presented,

        For example, 'Could you please give me the number of births with the midwife the most senior professional present between April and September 1995 inclusive' and not 'I understand the number of births with the midwife the most senior professional present are increasing. Is that so?'

7.   Diagnosing a problem involves linking the 'Cause and Effect'. By combining these together you should be able to identify why something is happening, or why it transpired in the first place.

A useful technique is to draw an outline of 'a fishbone' (Fig. 3.3).

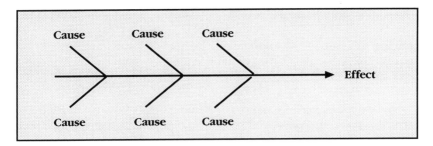

Fig. 3.3: Showing a framework that will link cause and effect.

The diagram can be completed as follows:

i)   Under 'Effect' - state the identified problem.
ii)   Next consider all the possible reasons why the problem occurred and enter each reason separately under 'Causes'.

For example, a problem occurred in the Obstetric theatre during the Christmas holiday period, when all the Caesarian section packs were used, and a member of the HSDU Department had to be called in to provide additional packs. Figure 3.4 shows there were six possible causes as to why the Obstetric theatre ran out of Caesarian section packs.

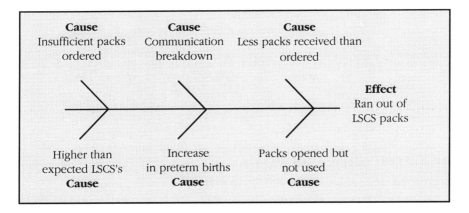

Fig. 3.4: Showing the possible causes as to why the LSCS packs ran out

8.   Despite using a basic model such as this it highlights just how complex it is to establish 'Cause and Effect'. The reason for this is because in the majority of cases problems are a result of more than one cause.

Therefore, it is necessary to examine all the possible reasons that could contribute to the problem before reaching a final conclusion.

9. 'Cause and Effect' is of little benefit for analysing 'circular problems' (Drummond, 1991). For example, when there is a personality clash it is irrelevant who started the conflict, because each person will continue to antagonize the other.

10. Having collected all the information, the final decision must be reconciled with the resources that are available. Questions such as 'will standards be maintained', and will 'the most cherished values survive?' (Schurr, 1968).

Schurr illustrates the importance of retaining values by providing a true account of an administrator with considerable ability, who employed all the scientific tools of management and among them carried out a work-study of the portering system. Although the staff cooperated to the best of their ability, some felt all was not well. They were at a loss to know exactly what was wrong until one day a student nurse asked a simple question: 'Why,' she asked, 'don't the porters whistle anymore?' The creation of an efficient organization is not enough - it must also be human.

11. When making the final decision there is a need not to be hurried. Having come to a conclusion you will be expected to stand by your decision, and this will take courage.

To help your final decision-making process the following principles are worth remembering:

- give yourself a period of quietness for reflection when making important decisions.
- try not to reach a conclusion at the end of a busy day or when you are considering another problem.
- circumstances can look very different after a 'nights sleep'.

12. Ultimately everything that you decide towards 'goal accomplishment' for the Maternity Services and the NHS Trust should according to La Monica (1994) be based on a conscious identified strategy that has the highest probability of success.

Using a scientific model
Vroom and Yetton's Contingency Model
The research of Vroom and Yetton in 1973 (La Monica, 1994) suggests there are various styles and circumstances when decision-making is more likely to succeed, and also circumstances when a particular approach is contra-indicated.

Their model is based on five leadership styles, arranged along a continuum from authoritarian to highly participative. By taking each of the five styles and using a diagram which represents a 'Decision Tree', managers can be facilitated in deciding which style is more appropriate to the situation being considered.

The management decisions styles with their individual interpretations for use are as follows:

1. The *Autocratic* Style - you decide to carry out the decision-making process yourself, based on the information you already have in your possession.

2. The *Research* Style - you obtain any necessary information from others, your boss, subordinates etc. and then make the decision yourself. You may or may not tell the others why you want the information.

3. The *Consultative* Style - you share the problem with others, your boss, subordinates etc. on an individual basis, obtaining their ideas and suggestions without bringing them together as a group. You will then make the decision, and it may or may not reflect the influence of the others.

4. The *Sharing* Style - you share the problem with others as a group, gathering the group's ideas and suggestions. You then make the decision yourself; it may or not be influenced by the group.

5. The *Consensus* Style - you share the problem with a group of affected people. You discuss with the group the problem and attempt to reach a consensus. You make no attempt to influence the group and you readily accept and implement their decision.

Deciding which approach to adopt

By using the 'Decision Tree' seven characteristics of the situation are considered, and plotted along the various branches. In this way, you can help yourself decide which of the five styles to adopt.

The characteristics

a) Quality: Is there a quality requirement? Could one solution be better than another? Is it important that the decision should be the right one?

b) Information: Do you have enough information yourself to make a good decision?

c) Problem structure: Is the problem structured? A structured problem is based on 'objective information' whereas an unstructured problem is a value judgement and can be subjective. Do you know exactly what information is needed, who possesses it and how to obtain it?

d) Acceptance: Is acceptance of the decision by others, e.g. midwives and users of the service, critical to implementation? Do they have to do anything towards solving the problem?

e) Prior probability of acceptance: If the decision was to be made by yourself in isolation are you fairly certain it would be accepted by others staff and users?

f)   Goal congruence: Do others - users of the service, the staff, the boss, medical colleagues, senior managers, Trust Board, purchasers - share the 'goals' to be obtained in solving the problem? Will they benefit if the problem is resolved?

g)   Difference of opinion: Is there likely to be conflict among other professionals and other members of the organization if the preferred solution is implemented?

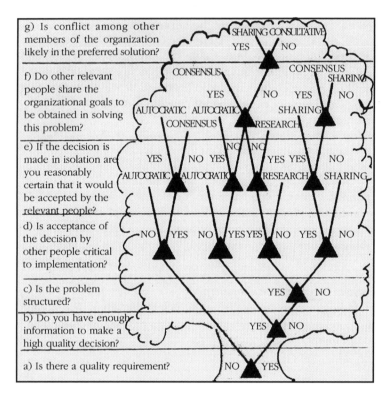

Fig 3.5: The 'Decision Tree' (Adapted from Stevensons, 1987)

Depending on whether the answer is 'yes' or 'no' to each of the above questions, some decision-making styles can be ruled out, and others are clearly more likely to lead to good decision-making. If you do not have enough information to make a good decision, or you consider that acceptance by the staff is critical but they are unlikely to accept a decision without consulting them, then the autocratic style is not suitable. If you consider that the staff cannot be relied on to make a decision in the best interests of the Maternity Services, without putting their own interests first, then the concensus style is not suitable.

There are some types of decision in which only one decision-style is likely to lead to a successful result, and there are others where more than one style is feasible and therefore likely to succeed. Although using the 'Decision Tree' is not a difficult exercise (Watkin, 1978) it does require the ability to think logically.

Application of the 'Decision Tree' model to a maternity services situation

MIDWIFERY CASE EXAMPLE

You are the midwifery manager responsible for introducing a new system of tape-recorded handover in the labour suite. This was your idea and you felt you had the full cooperation of the midwives. You had briefed them and provided education and training prior to implementation, and they seemed happy to go ahead. Recently you have become aware that the new arrangement is not working, and the midwives have reverted to the old system of report-handover.

How are you going to resolve this situation, and which management style ate you going to adopt? By using the Decision Tree model (Fig. 3.5), the best management style for solving this problem can be decided. The result is shown in Figure 3.6.

Resulting Style		Consensus	
f) Do others share the goals to be obtained in solving the problem?	YES	YES	
e) If the decision was made in isolation would it be accepted by others?	NO		NO
d) Is acceptance by others critical to implementation?	YES	YES	
c) Is the problem structured? Does it have objectives?	YES		YES
b) Do you have enough information to make good decisions?	NO		NO
a) Is there a quality assessment?	YES	YES	

Fig. 3.6: Using the 'Decision Tree' to resolve the midwifery case example.

If subsequently you do develop a routine of analysing important decisions by using 'Vroom and Yetton's' Scientific Model, there is still no guarantee that your decision-making will be the right one. But at least it will help you avoid the elementary mistake of making decisions autocratically, and without the relevant information. Moreover, it will help you avoid using a participative decision-making style, if there is any chance a group of staff will come up with a decision you may not be able to accept for the Maternity Services. Further more, an experimental study by Vroom and Jago in 1978 (La Monica, 1994) suggests that managers who use the Decision Tree model have more effective outcomes and acceptance by staff than those who do not use the model.

Stevenson (1987) in her summing up on the use of Scientific Models, is cautious about assuming that models based on American or Industrial experience are automatically applicable to the National Health Service. She considers 'Vroom's Model' has three shortcomings:

- it assumes all decisions are discrete, whereas in the NHS a problem is not always clear or so easily defined.

- it assumes all managers are able to vary their approach, whereas Stevenson found in reality NHS managers tended to use one style.

- it omits some of the other options available for decision-making in the NHS.

She does conclude, however, that if managers are prepared to use Scientific Models and use them as a basis for their own models of decision-making adapted for NHS use, they might begin to find 'optimum' solutions as opposed to 'satisficing' solutions. A satisficing solution being defined by Simon in 1960 (Stevenson, 1987) as 'the adoption of the first satisfactory solution suggested - sacrificing the optimum for the convenient'.

Group decision-making

Decisions are sometimes made by groups, and often groups are consulted, either formally or informally, over decisions that have been proposed for local and national changes.

Handy (1993) believes effective groups, be they problem-solving or producing, are the ones that set themselves standards and have a maintenance programme in practice. He contends that groups where the leader does not get the group to set and adopt standards, will satisfy at the lowest level as far as decision-making is concerned.

Also, there is the question of whether groups should make decisions at all, because of the way groups behave and function. When a decision is made by a group, is it totally reliable? What was the process used to agree the decision? Was it made through harmonious decision-making or coercion? Effective decision-making requires all views to be articulated and debated seriously (Drummond, 1991). Everyone in the group should be encouraged to contribute and each of their contributions should be properly considered by all members.

To consider whether group decision-making is reliable, first it is necessary to understand how groups form, and the behaviour of people in groups - this is known as 'group dynamics'.

Understanding group dynamics

A group is more than just a collection of people. Each group has a particular identity which is unique, and this will influence the behaviour of individuals in the group. Members may:

- behave differently in a group than they do as an individual
- behave differently in different groups.

A group exists for a reason, and to achieve the purpose of its existence the members of the group are required to communicate and interact with one another. As interactions occur, members become aware of each other, and feelings and emotions are exchanged. With the exchange of emotions and a shared incentive, gradually members become aware of their need for each other and start to see themselves as a group. As soon as a group is formed disparities emerge. Some members talk more than others, some get actively involved while others remain passive, and some members become forceful and powerful.

People occupy different positions within a group. 'Pecking-orders' may emerge in accordance with respective status i.e. a midwifery sister may automatically assume the role as leader whereas the newly qualified midwife may assume the role as 'minute-taker'.

The leader of a group is powerful - she or he is at the centre of communications. A danger is that a leader may presuppose power because of this central position. More seriously a leader could become dominant, and dictate the group's agenda, block communications and misinterpret information. This would distort and impair the group's decision-making process.

Group decisions are often influenced more by who is speaking than what is actually being said. This type of power corrupts.

Should groups make decisions?

It has been shown in experimental studies (Handy, 1993) that groups who attack a problem systematically perform better than groups who muddle through, or evolve. The performance of the group will be influenced by the kind of standards they adopt, and how each member is encouraged to participate.

Handy believes there are neglected resources in groups, which may be due to:

- opposing factions - and it is the responsibility of the leader to help members to manage and resolve their conflict, and come to a compromise

- members not listening to each other - therefore the leader must clarify and summarize so there is a common awareness of what has been said, before the decision-making process can begin.

As far as the decision-making process itself is concerned this is of crucial importance, as a decision will be made by either:

- authority - with the leader making the decision or forcing a decision on the group

- majority vote, very rarely by minority vote. The problem with this type of decision-making is that pressure tactics may be used by one or more of the members to achieve a majority

- consensus - which is a psychological state where members of the group see rationale in the decision, agree and support it.

It is a fact that most group decisions are negative-decisions and as such often pass unnoticed as decisions.

According to Drummond (1991) generally groups are counter-productive where decisions require:

• speed
• careful concentration
• sustained thought.

Where they are of value is in their capacity to generate ideas and alternatives, supply solutions to specific problems, and to provide views, responses and comments on Consultative Proposal documents. The real merit of a group such as this, is that members bring together their experiences, skills and qualifications from various backgrounds. Rather than the group being entrusted with a final decision, it is better that they are asked for their views, to identify options, or make comments upon proposals.

How to deal with crisis decision-making

Although crisis management is best avoided, in reality serious problems do arise suddenly and have to be dealt with immediately. Usually this is because smaller problems have not been recognized or they have been ignored, and have not been appropriately dealt with.

The best approach is to have your own personal technique for dealing with crises as they occur. Develop a checklist and keep it accessible, so you can refer to it at such times. Remember when a crisis occurs you need to respond calmly but urgently.

Handling a crisis involves:

• identifying and defining what the problem is - alone or with others
• stating the desired result
• making a list of possible solutions
• testing the suitability of these solutions
• choosing the preferred solution
• implementing action without delay.

Summary

Effective decision-making is about formulating events, bringing about results and modelling the future. Ineffective decision-making includes 'decisive inaction' which thwarts change, and making reactive 'decisionless-decisions' which deal with the short-term only. Escalation and entrapment result from short-planned decisions and cause decision-makers to become trapped in 'loosing courses of action'.

The three main types of decision-making relevant to maternity services management are strategic, operational and personal-professional.

Management decision theory derives from the early economists and proceeds from the assumption that decision-makers are motivated to maximize profit and situations. Rationality in decision-making is essential. A midwifery manager may consider herself to be totally objective but it is virtually impossible to prevent others trying to manipulate the decision-making process for their own ends. An awareness of this is essential.

There are various models and techniques to help midwifery managers with decision-making. The traditional Synoptic Model provides a logical framework for identifying problems and for prioritizing goals and options prior to implementing a change. The use of such a model avoids intuition and irrationality in decision-making. Despite its simple framework the Synoptic Model is not easy to use, mainly because decision-making is in itself involved and complicated.

A fundamental part of the decision-making process is the accumulation of the correct information. Methodical information gathering and the use of the 'cause and effect technique' are useful procedures to assist the decision-making process. The scientific model of Vroom and Yetton is an effective model for deciding the most suitable management style for solving a problem.

Whether groups should make decisions is debatable. Groups that set themselves standards are more able, but because of the way groups behave can a decision always be reliable? The group decision-making process can range from consensus to coercion. If a leader presupposes power this can distort the decision-making process. Usually groups are counter-productive when decisions require speed and concentration, but good for generating ideas and providing views and comments.

Crisis decision-making is best avoided, but in reality serious problems can occur suddenly and have to be dealt with immediately. The best approach for dealing with crises is to have a pre-planned personal technique, which is accessible and up to date.

CHAPTER FOUR

The Challenge of Change

*'We must learn individually and as organizations to welcome change
and innovation as vigorously as we have fought it in the past'*
(Tom Peters, 1990)

As we move towards the 21st century in a constantly changing National Health Service, midwifery managers and midwifery sisters will be required to be competent at managing change. In addition to regular reviews of clinical practice, getting the most suitable organizational structure and monitoring the efficiency and effectiveness of staff, opportunities for innovations in maternity care have never been greater, particularly with the requirements of the recommendations of the *Patients Charter* (1991, 1995) and *Changing Childbirth* (1993). The capacity to innovate change promptly is emerging as the criterion for survival (Harding, 1988) and consequently strategies that are capable of flexibility and adaptability will assume a greater significance than ever before. Unfortunately, change is often badly handled, and resistance by staff to change is often neglected or ignored. The ability to introduce change with a minimal amount of resistance is a key managerial skill.

According to Pearson and Thomas (1991) there are five major issues in the management of change:

1.   The difficulty in identifying all the problems that are likely to arise during the change-process.
2.   Estimating the amount of time needed to deal with all the difficulties and to persuade people to accept the change.
3.   The frequent lack of commitment to the change - 'the change is desired by "them" not "us"'.
4.   The impact of new crises during the change process which often means a further change in direction.
5.   The total time it takes for the whole change process to be undertaken.

One of the permanent features of our lives is change (Walton,1988). Most people generally accept that the needs of each individual will change over time, so why do so many staff expect, or want to behave as if all around them is static and time has 'stood still'? Naturally people react to change in different ways, but generally human-beings are creatures of habit with a tendency to protect the familiar, and thus have an inclination to resist change. At work its very easy to get caught up in routines, i.e. ward-routines, carrying out procedures in the way we have always done them, and continually conducting meetings in the same format. So often the circumstances that made procedures and actions necessary in the first place have altered, and yet there is still a tendency to carry on as before.

There are no short cuts to implementing change. The best way for those managing change is to approach the whole issue as a process of learning, by understanding how people react to change, developing a deeper knowledge of how organizations work and by using the many techniques and methods available to facilitate the change-process.

Reaction to change

People respond or react to change in different ways, and this may be dependent on whether the change is temporary or permanent. For example:

- a change in the pattern of work in a postnatal ward as a result of a brief period of staff sickness will require short-term adjustment. This arrangement would be considered temporary and consequently staff would be more inclined to support and accept this change.

- a permanent reduction of the staff establishment in the postnatal ward would be a different matter, and would require a major review of staff utilization in the ward. This arrangement would be seen as permanent and staff would be more inclined to reject this change.

Usually staff who feel a change has been imposed upon them will respond less positively than staff who have been actively involved in reviewing and initiating a change.

Resistance to change, despite what many people believe, can be both good and bad. It can be viewed in two ways:

- good - that which maintains order and stability
- bad - that which effectively hinders and blocks change.

Therefore, it can be seen that resistance to change can be used as a valuable balancing and accommodating technique, which could prevent a midwifery manager going headlong into a situation without prior or proper planning. Through staff asking questions, and challenging a proposed change, the original plans may need to be revised. This would result in a more successful implementation because the staff feel they have been more involved in the final decision.

On the other hand resistance can be corrupt. This is when it is used to prevent or block something which may be essential or advantageous to mothers and babies, the staff or the organization.

Why do people resist change?

Not all changes are resisted. Although staff may be inclined to oppose change, this is sometimes counteracted by the likely rewards associated with the change, or an opportunity of a new experience. For example, salary increases are generally welcomed but where the change involves a change in personal working conditions or in interpersonal relationships, reactions are likely to occur.

Resistance to change is usually to the way the manager introduces the change, rather than to the change itself (Hunt, 1983). Where change is threatened, often it is the meaning of the word 'change' which provokes the resistance, as its interpretation often becomes distorted due to poor communication. According to La Monica (1994) just the term 'change agent' can arouse defensiveness in the subjects of change and can threaten the agent.

It was Toffler in 1971 (Boot, Cowling and Stanworth, 1982) who described change as 'a roaring current' that 'overturns institutions, shifts our values and shrivels our lives'. This can be better understood if we accept the view of Hunt (1983) that organizations are not designed for each individual, and thus individual goals can never be completely satisfied in an organization.

It is, therefore, not remarkable that on a personal level change can generate fear. To most people change is full of doubts, uncertainties and often mistrust. Even if a member of staff can see that a change would be an improvement on the current situation, there is still doubt about their personal involvement and how the change will effect them. Questions such as:

- why do we need to change?
- what is wrong with the way we are doing it now?
- will I have to change my job?
- will I have to move to another ward or department?
- will I have to learn new skills?
- will my position and status change?
- what is in it for me?
- when will the change happen?
- what future is planned for my ward or department?
- who will my new midwifery manager be?
- can I trust the new management arrangements?

If these questions are left unanswered, staff tend to internalize their doubts. Not only is this unproductive, but it can be dangerous, as energy is focused on their own uncertainties instead of concentrating on the care of mothers and babies. Also staff in this situation are more inclined to share their distrust with other doubters, and this usually leads to group-resistance to the change. In 1985, Davis and Newstrom (La Monica, 1994) described this type of resistance as one based on emotion and selfish desires, where the benefits of the outcomes of a change are ignored because of their own personal needs and fears.

The degree of resistance depends on several factors:

1.   Feelings of inadequacy felt by the staff, and whether they sense they lack the power to bring about the change.

2.   How radical is the change, and how much different will it be from current procedures and practices, especially in relation to values and beliefs? For example, the introduction of a waterbirth service was for some midwives difficult to conceptualize and accept, despite additional education, training and revised policy.

3.   How much the staff hold on to old values and the way they have always done things.

4.   How much inconvenience will the change cause.

5.   How they perceive the manager implementing the change or the person they see as the 'change agent', with regard to their role, credibility and capability.

How resistance to change can be manifested

According to Vaughan and Pillmoor (1989) resistance is inherent in the change process, and they describe several classic ways in which resistance can be displayed. The kinds of behaviour which may occur are:

*   'Lip service' - this is when staff listen to suggestions and may even contribute their own ideas with the manager or 'change agent' present. Usually they have no intention of changing and when they are required to act they are not prepared to do anything.

*   Aggression - when staff are unhappy about a change it is not unusual for them to display aggressive behaviour. In some way this can be seen as a 'protective mechanism' to counteract their uncertainty and fear.

*   Destruction - this may occasionally occur when a staff member or a small group of staff rigorously try to put a stop to a change. Usually this is because the effects of the change may be threatening or unacceptable to them. Sometimes this behaviour is open, i.e. by vocal opposition to the change and gaining local support with other staff or through the media. At other times destructive behaviour may become evident in more subtle ways, i.e. giving sympathy rather than empathy, thus reinforcing feelings of self-pity which could destroy the commitment of staff to a planned change.

*   Lack of continuity - this is when staff appear to support a change but make excuses for not trying it out. For example 'we're busy today - but will do it another day when the ward is less busy.' and then 'we can't do it this week because we have two new student midwives starting in the ward.'

Gradually the excuses get weaker, and over a period of time this type of behaviour will undermine a change. Eventually the proposed change will disappear altogether and will be 'left on the shelf'.

Beating resistance to change

Change does not have to be a negative experience. One of the most successful ways to fight resistance to change is to first and foremost accept change is a natural process, that occurs in everyones life. It is the word 'change' that is the problem not the actual process of changing. La Monica (1994) calls the 'label of change the insidious wart' but considers the process of changing as simply cell regeneration which happens without cognitive awareness, with no one really feeling it. This view is supported by Mauksch and Miller (1981) who contend there is no longer a debate about whether or not change will occur, but at directing attention to diagnosing the speed, direction, and impact of change and how it might be controlled. They maintain that staff usually accept change will occur despite their own vested interests.

Today midwifery managers are being encouraged to pay more attention to their organization's 'corporate culture' when trying to manage change more effectively. We now see NHS Trusts concentrating on changing the culture of their business in a bid to improve performance. Developing a 'corporate culture' has been at the heart of the NHS reforms, but how much do managers and staff completely understand the meaning of 'corporate culture'?

Understanding the corporate culture

A helpful definition of corporate culture is 'the way we do things around here' (Pearson and Thomas, 1991).

What this seemingly simple yet profound statement reveals about an organization is its management style, its atmosphere and its ambience. Organizational culture is made up of:

1. Beliefs and values
2. Norms
3. Style

1. Beliefs and values: that the staff have about their organization, and where it belongs locally, nationally and universally. How the staff feel about their own NHS Trust and where they believe it stands world-wide in providing high standards of health care. For example, staff in the Maternity Services would be heard to say: 'I believe this Maternity Service stands for quality', 'I consider we are the leaders in providing partnership in care' and 'I think we are always striving to be the best'.

2. Norms: the usual behaviour of those working and using an organization. The behaviour which is generally most comfortable and acceptable, and therefore endorsed by the staff as 'norm'. For example, in the Maternity Services:

- the usual approach to solving problems and decision-making
- the way meetings are arranged and conducted
- the use of first names when caring for mothers and their family
- how clinical standards are set and measured.

3. Style: the management style and the accepted behaviour in the organization. This will reflect the way managers operate throughout the NHS Trust, from the Chief Executive and the Board of Directors to those managing the service and providing care in the wards and departments. For example, the management style of midwifery managers:

- is open door
- is through leadership and empowering staff
- is autocratic
- is through the use of rewards and punishments.

To understand organizational culture further a useful technique is to consider 'Norms and Style' as being above the surface of the organization, and 'Beliefs and Values' as being below (Fig. 4.1).

> Above the surface - Norms and Style
>
> Below the surface - Beliefs and Values

Fig.4.1: Showing the organizational culture

With regard to 'Beliefs and values' it is always difficult to know what staff really think about the organization for which they work, let alone getting them to articulate these thoughts. On the other hand it is fairly easy to distinguish an organization's management style, by observing the way managers go about their business, and by monitoring the standards and quality of care that is achieved. These tell us a great deal about the culture of an organization.

For example, how does a NHS Trust deal with problems?

- does it appoint a multi-disciplinary team or delegate an appropriate individual manager to solve the problem?
- how does the Maternity Service conduct its meetings? Are they open participative meetings to which all staff are invited to attend or meetings that are closed and secretive?

Culture is something that modern managers must concern themselves with. Sooner or later an organization is assessed by its performance in the market place, and NHS Trusts are no exception. How a Trust is perceived is the critical issue. Its image is mainly created by the behaviour of its staff as well as its performance. Purchasers, customers, users, suppliers, competitors and the media all have a perception of a NHS

Trust. This perception is produced in many ways. With regard to Maternity Services, on one level it may be the way midwives welcome mothers to their first antenatal clinic, or the way telephonists answer the phone. On another it may be the quality of individual care each mother receives, and their subsequent level of satisfaction on completion of that care. Or whether accounts are submitted promptly to purchasers and whether accurate statistics are provided regularly. Or the way in which staff respond to consumer-representatives i.e. visits of members of the Maternity Services Liaison Committee, the Community Health Council and the media. All these interactions with the 'outside world' will give a perception of the Trust's Maternity Services.

Perception is formed by behaviour, which will ultimately determine whether the Trust or a sub-speciality within the NHS Trust i.e. Maternity Services, is profitable or not, and whether it has an advantage over other Trusts. As far as performance is concerned, Pearson and Thomas (1991) consider culture can be both an accelerator and a brake, and they illustrate this point clearly with the model (Fig. 4.2), developed by Colin Waterhouse of Price Waterhouse.

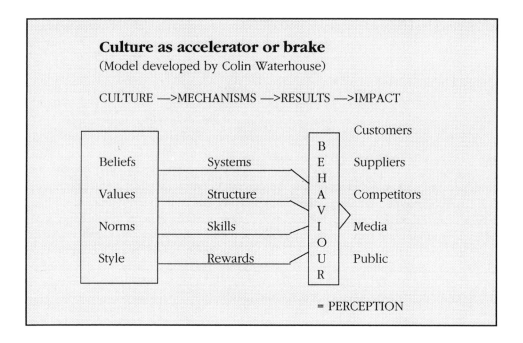

Fig. 4.2: Model to show culture can be seen as an accelerator or brake
(Reprinted by kind permission of Harper Collins Publishers from Pearson, B., Thomas, N. (1991).*The Shorter MBA.*)

According to Handy (1993) cultural confusion is one of the principal ills that plaque an organization. It shows up when assessing efficiency or more clearly in what he calls *slack*, - requiring extra resources, taking longer to produce the services and working extra hours. Slack he says is 'the organization's balm used to ease the pain of inefficiency. It is management's easy option and a way of cushioning a wrong culture.'

Managers can influence the behaviour of staff by using the following:

- Systems - by investing in information technology this will reduce costs and improve efficiency. It is predicted that by providing managers with up-to-date financial, clinical and resource information this will enable them to make more effective and speedier decisions, which in turn will improve the overall performance and business in a NHS Trust.

- Structure - by developing the most appropriate management structure for managing the clinical specialities and the business of a NHS Trust. Currently the de-centralized flattened structure is favoured, where the power is shared more evenly and more control is given to those directly involved in clinical care. Fashions will change and debates will continue as to which structure - centralized, decentralized or divisional - is the best for the Trust. Indeed structures will frequently be altered in an attempt to change the behaviour of the staff and improve performance.

- Skills - the willingness and the ability of staff to practice competently, maintain high professional standards and develop new skills is central to providing a quality health service. In-service education and training updates staff on current research and methods of practice but it also encourages them to do things differently. Thus a major objective of in-service training is to affect a change in the behaviour of staff and improve performance.

- Rewards - by changing and improving pay and conditions of service, and providing reward-packages, i.e. free beverages, cafeteria benefits, the intention is towards changing the behaviour of staff. Also, towards improving performance. For example, performance related pay is aimed at improving the quality and output, and incentive schemes are aimed at increasing the number of operations carried out and securing more contracts.

Often these 'mechanisms' work but frequently they fail to produce the required behaviour changes. The reason is usually that senior management have failed to consider the impact of the changes on the organization's culture. It is a fact that very little culture change will occur unless there is a commitment and an understanding of the changes by senior management.

Changing the organizational culture

There is no right or wrong culture but the culture must match the NHS Trusts strategic plan.

Changing a Trust's culture is not an easy task, it takes years rather than months to affect a lasting change. Likewise creating the right culture for the Maternity Services will take time and energy, even with the help and support of such reports as *Changing Childbirth* (1993). In truth, creating the right culture is a continuous process, as it must be ensured that the culture always matches the Maternity Services strategy.

The essential requirements for a successful culture change in Maternity Services are:

1.   A clear vision and a definite sense of direction - of what the Maternity Service wants to achieve and where it wants to be in the future.

2.   A commitment to the change by the Trust Management Board and those managing the Maternity Services, and an acceptance and ownership by the staff providing maternity care.

3.   Managers and staff working consistently together, by recognizing and applauding innovations and change, but at the same time being ready and prepared for any setbacks.

4.   An effective communications programme emphasizing the role of managers and of the staff in the change process. This will secure commitment and ownership of the changes.

The change process

This was first defined and discussed by Lewin in 1951 (Walton, 1988) and later by Schein in 1968 (Boot, Cowling and Stanworth, 1982).

Basically change consists of three progressive stages, and each stage needs to be worked through before moving to the next. The stages are:

•   Unfreezing: This involves breaking down the usual way people do things. It includes interrupting and breaking down normal routines and customs, so that staff are ready to accept new alternatives. As the title 'unfreezing' suggests the forces that act on an individual are 'thawed' or 'melted down'.

     This phase is crucial for the midwifery manager and takes the most time as it involves externally motivating the staff towards the desired goal.

•   Changing: Once people are motivated to change they are ready to accept new patterns of behaviour in one of three ways:
     - compliance: through rewards or punishments
     - identification: associating closely with role models
     - internalization: having an' intrinsic urge to change

•   Refreezing: This occurs when new behaviours become part of a person's personality, when they have knowledge, positive attitudes and experience of the new behaviours. These new behaviours must be positively reinforced after the change has occurred to ensure continued 'refreezing'.

How to manage change

•   Cultivate an environment conducive to change - If changes are frequent and you manage these effectively with successful results, they will become more acceptable. Staff will get used to the idea of change, and begin to welcome change as a normal aspect of their work. This in turn will encourage ideas for change to be generated from the staff themselves, and you can then involve them in planning, implementing and evaluating these changes.

- Create a belief in management - Much will depend on the degree of confidence and trust the staff have in you as a manager and or 'change agent'. To accomplish successful change you will need to build up 'trust' with the staff through leadership, good communications, sound working relationships, teamworking and empowering the staff.

- Get the timing right - You must take time in introducing change, in creating a cordial and receptive atmosphere, and giving staff time to get used to an idea before starting to implement. Occasionally there may be a few situations when a quick introduction to change without prior notice will work, but these are usually associated with short temporary changes.

- Provide information - You must provide staff with accurate information, giving them details about the change and why it is required. Emphasis should be on the benefits of the change i.e. the advantages to the mothers and babies, and how the midwives can gain from the change too.

- Emphasize the benefits - Proposals for change have a greater chance of being acted on if you can show there are benefits for the 'principal components'. The more overlap between the users, individuals and the organization (Fig. 4.3) the more likely there is to be a successful change-process.

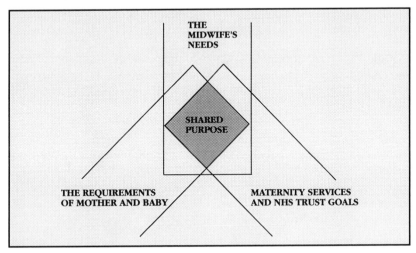

Fig. 4.3 The shared purpose of users, individuals and the organization

- Avoid confrontations - This is sometimes difficult, but it is important for you to encourage the staff to adhere to the basics, and concentrate on the positive aspects of the change. Fault-finding by criticising the past is of little value, it is best to try and direct all energy towards a desire to make progress towards the change.

- Do not expect instant support - The first step is to gain the cooperation of the staff and get them to participate in the decision-making about the change. Once you have achieved this they will feel more committed towards the decision to change.

  Informing staff about a change increases their awareness, but involving them in participative and mutual decision-making is more likely to result in acceptance and 'ownership' and further commitment to the decision.

- Progress towards an agreeable conclusion - Your aim is to get as many staff as possible to accept and support the change, not for a hundred per cent shift. Once the 'believers' are openly committed to implementing the change, usually peer-group pressure will influence the 'doubters' and 'non believers' and gradually you will gain more support.

- Provide an opportunity for questions and discussion - You must give staff the chance to ask questions and the opportunity for discussion, particularly on areas of agreement. Unanswered questions can lead to uncertainty about the change, personal anxieties and distrust in your management ability and style.

  Problems and objections should be listened to with understanding, but always bear in mind that what you are being told may not necessarily be the real reason for the objection. Sometimes members of staff will hide reasons for rejecting a change which they do not want to admit even to themselves.

- Give credit for the change - Staff who have been involved with a change should be given a share of the credit. Always acknowledge publicly their contribution and involvement.

- Provide in-Service education - When further education, additional training or retraining is required to implement the change this must be provided. You must also emphasize to the staff that continued help and support will be available to them during and after the change.

- Agree and plan a programme and timetable - As soon as you feel there is reasonable agreement between you and the staff, immediately draw up a plan of action so as to keep up the 'momentum for change'. Put together a programme and timetable, give this to the staff involved and disseminate widely. Don't forget to send copies to your Clinical Director, and other senior managers such as directors of the Trust Board for information.

- Evaluate the change-process - Get the staff who have been involved in the change-process to evaluate whether the change has been implemented correctly and the goals met. This can be done by discussion, observation, structured interviews, questionnaires and reports.

  Results of these findings should be shared with the staff, your boss and senior managers and where appropriate users and purchasers of maternity services. As

Mathieson and Kellet (1994) remind us 'learning and progress take time'. It is through planning, implementing and sustaining changes that anxiety levels will eventually fall and confidence grows. It is only then that staff will see the benefits of change, feel energized and empowered.

Force Field analysis

Force Field analysis is a planning tool that midwifery managers can use to help analyse events and problems from an action point of view. The tool is developed from a systems approach to problems and is credited to Kurt Lewin (1951) whose 'field theory' described a field of forces or pressures acting on a specific event at any particular time. It is based on the notion that all situations can be seen in temporary equilibrium i.e. the forces acting to change a situation are balanced by the forces acting to resist the change. This can be depicted as a simple diagram as in Figure 4.4.

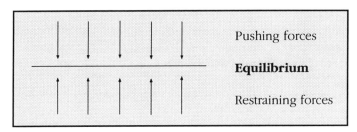

Fig 4.4: Showing the pushing and restraining forces of change

This view of events is a dynamic one, which acknowledges temporariness in all things. It is viewed from a moderately existential standpoint that 'man' is free and responsible for 'his' acts. It offers midwifery managers an opportunity to see situations as being potentially changeable, if they can first identify the 'pushing and restraining forces' and then endeavour to change their direction and strength.

La Monica (1994) has taken 'Force Field Analysis' and adapted it to a useful technique for understanding what is happening when a manager wishes to move a system from Actual to Optimal. She contends that by using the Force Field Analysis concept 'the difference' between Actual and Optimal' can be explained.

Using La Monica's method the following case example of a problem can be defined:

• Actual: Midwives are being late, and frequently do not attend to present Parent Education classes for which they are scheduled.

• Optimal: Midwives who are scheduled to present Parent Education classes make these their overall priority, arrive in adequate time to prepare for the class and do not cancel.

• Problem: Midwives arrive late or cancel their attendance to present previously arranged Parent Education classes.

- Goal: To have midwives arrive in good time to present Parent Education classes and do not have to cancel their attendance.

In this case the midwifery manager or midwifery sister would want to move Actual to Optimal and to accomplish the Goal. This process can be accomplished by movement as seen in Figure 4.5.

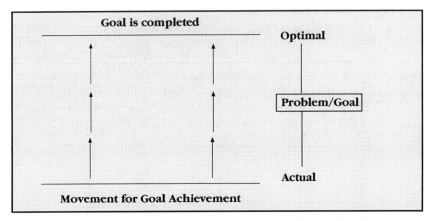

Fig. 4.5: Movement for goal achievement (reproduced with kind permission of Macmillan Press from La Monica, 1994)

With Force Field analysis we are required to imagine that the line symbolizing the Goal is suspended between the forces that are working towards moving the actual to optimal known as the Pushing or Driving forces - and the forces that are working against the move from actual to optimal - known as the Restraining forces.

To facilitate the use of this process La Monica advises us to imagine that weights Figure 4.6 can be added to either side of the imaginary line to portray the relative importance to each force.

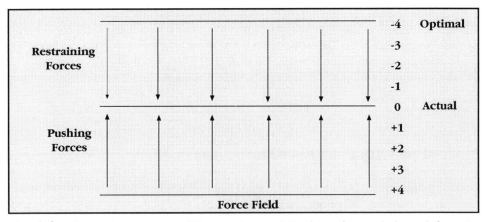

Fig. 4.6: Relative importance of Restraining and Pushing forces (adapted from La Monica, 1994)

If an equal amount of Pushing and Restraining forces are operative in the Field there is no movement to the Actual line, and this is described as a state of equilibrium. But if the Pushing forces outweigh the Restraining forces there would be a shift towards the Optimal.

Thus a manager can accomplish change by increasing or augmenting the Pushing forces, or alternatively by eliminating or suppressing the Restraining forces. In either case the Actual would move towards the Optimal line.

Below is a Force field analysis using the case example of midwives arriving late, or cancelling their attendance, when scheduled to present Parent Education classes (Fig. 4.7).

In this example the Pushing forces are equal to the Restraining forces. Therefore the Midwifery manager can concentrate on either group of forces, or on both groups to bring about change. It is, however, best to develop the positive forces, as this will make the negative forces appear less significant.

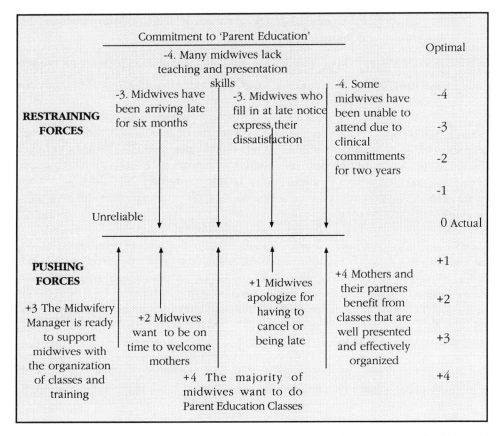

Fig. 4.7: Showing the pushing and restraining forces in the case example (adapted from La Monica, 1994)

The problem still has to be analysed, with the midwifery manager deciding on the best solution(s) to achieve the ultimate goal. Thus it can be seen that Force Field analysis is a good tool for providing the midwifery manager with items to focus on for the solution phase of problem-solving. Focusing on the forces with the highest weights usually has the biggest impact on affecting change.

Conflict theory in change management

Occasionally changes occur without people being fully aware that something has changed until after it has actually happened e.g. the government changes such as 'The Abortion Act' (1967) and 'The Health of the Nation' (1992). According to Olson (Mauksch and Miller, 1981) this is not usually the norm. He contends that most social changes are preceded by conflicting forces seeking to prevent change.

Clearly conflict is not a necessary or sufficient condition for change, but there is substantial evidence that conflict promotes change. For example:

•   staff who complain that their on-call arrangements are unsatisfactory enforce the midwifery manager to undertake a review, which could subsequently result in a change and improve the arrangements.

•   a protest to the finance department by midwifery managers and midwives complaining that the insurance cover for lease cars is insufficient, would result in a change and improved cover.

Forces outside an organization can also be a source of conflict that result in changes being made within an organization. A good example of this occurred during the 1980s, when a minority of mothers joined with members of the National Childbirth Trust and objected to routine induction of labour. Eventually this forced a review of routine induction procedures and the practice was discontinued, with a more flexible, individual approach taking its place.

The Conflict theory of social change contends that at the basis of most organizational change is some form of conflict which is experienced by staff. Members of staff, in an effort to resolve or remove conflict, work to change certain circumstances within the organization. Their attempts to change behaviour and conditions usually put them into conflict with other groups who do not encounter similar conflicts. Also some groups may have reasons why they want to resist the proposed change. It can be brought about as follows:

1.   A group of staff in conflict attempt to alter or change a situation, so that the conflict (this can also be described as frustration, confusion, discord, insecurity) will be reduced or removed.

2.   Conflict may be caused as a result of a proposed or attempted change in the organization. There are staff who have a vested interest in keeping the situation as it is. For example, professionals - midwives, consultant medical staff, radiologists - may want to maintain the 'status quo'. A group of midwives may

have an interest in keeping their conditions of service the same to protect themselves from loss of income, reputation or status.

3.   Because one group of professional staff are dissatisfied and want change, it does not mean that their proposed change is always in the best interest of the whole organization. Extreme coercion to change in these circumstances could result in the breakdown of the organization itself.

4.   Different values, beliefs and attitudes between various groups of staff within an organization are also a reason for conflict over proposed and actual change. For example, some midwives believe team midwifery provides more direct personal care for mothers and babies, whilst others believe the traditional approach is more personalized.

5.   A group of staff who want to change some aspects of an organization's order may produce conflict from other staff members, especially those who prefer to go on in the same way and do not want to change.

Although conflict can promote change, change is only one of several possible outcomes of conflict. In severe situations of conflict, for example - where staff are involved in gross disobedience or their action is a deliberate disruption to patient care - the outcome could result in disciplinary action or dismissal.

Strategies and tactics for implementing change in midwifery

Midwifery managers and midwives who want to successfully implement change in the workplace, must first devise a work plan. Successful implementation of a change is not usually achieved without it being carefully 'thought through' and planned in advance.

To overcome 'normal' resistance to change, strategies and tactics need to be incorporated. These are defined as follows:

*   strategy - a master plan of action
*   tactics - activities for implementing a strategy
*   tactic - an activity planned and designed to carry out a part of the plan and aimed at implementing change.

Thus a strategy can consist of a number of tactics. Strategies and tactics will vary depending on the circumstances for the change, and the setting where the change is to take place.

Identifying goals

In order to implement a strategy it is necessary to first identify the type of goal required.

There are two main types:

- Long-range goal - this is usually one of such magnitude that its achievement requires a number of sophisticated strategies. These would have to be detailed and diverse to allow for consultation with staff and for their responses prior to the actual process of implementation.

- Short-range goal - this usually has few if any permanent implications and requires much less preparation and different tactics.

Achieving the 'Changing Childbirth' recommendations

Strategies for implementing such an immense change as *Changing Childbirth* will take a long time, as will their implementation. Developing goals for a change of such magnitude - one which is certain to revolutionize maternity care in this country - will require careful planning and participation by everyone involved. There are no short cuts to implementing such a macro-level change.

Strategies for implementing the recommendations of *Changing Childbirth* must first be directed towards the NHS Trust directors, working closely with the Clinical Director for Maternity and Neonatal Services, the midwifery manager(s), the service manager and midwives. The Trust will need to give agreement on the levels of management involved, what resources are required and the plans to be used to develop the change process.

Strategies such as these have diplomatic and political overtones (Mauksch and Miller, 1981). To implement the recommendations of *Changing Childbirth* there will be numbers of people (staff) who will have to be persuaded and influenced by effective strategies and tactics.

Getting the target population, the group that will be most personally and significantly affected by the change, to acknowledge and accept the need for change is the biggest challenge. In *Changing Childbirth* midwives are a large target population, but not only midwives. Also involved are hospital doctors, general practitioners, professions allied to medicine, support workers, in fact everyone who has direct and indirect contact with mothers and babies.

To implement change successfully requires not only acceptance and approval but also enthusiasm on the part of the target population. Effective communication is critical, because if the target population believes it has not been consulted appropriately it will become negative, or at worst resistant or obstructive.

The best strategy for winning over a target group is:

- find out what the different members of the target group know about the proposed change(s)

- what attitudes do they have towards the recommendations for change.

Once these are known, then tactics can be used to persuade the target group that the changes are beneficial and acceptable. Tactics that can be used are:

- providing information, inducements, incentives, rewards
- providing education, training and development.

Accomplishing change in the maternity services without conflict and resistance

Conflict or resistance to change reflect the climate of the organization. Is it one that is conducive to resolving conflict or not? A Maternity Service that has an attitude of smoothing over conflicts in an attempt to avoid facing the basic issues in the change process will not be susceptible to change. Organizations in which conflicts rarely occur usually have effective communication systems and, because the resolution to conflict is constructively managed, do not fear these conflicts.

'Avoiding conflict at any cost is as unproductive as the artificial creation of conflict' (Mauksch and Miller, 1989). Conflict and resistance to change are a part of everyday behaviour.

Tactics that can be used in conflict situations:

- Levelling - an honest approach to the issues involved. Looking at things as they are perceived by others and openly attempting their resolution, solution and conclusion.

- Control - as soon as a conflict arises the midwifery manager will use the power of control in an attempt to resolve it, exercising authority as a means of control.

- Denial - the least helpful tactic for resolution. When conflict is denied, the midwifery manager has to be realistic about how to deal with the denial. Accepting the person's denial and believing nothing can be done is not productive. Conflict will not just go away, and consequently will not lead to successful change.

Other tactics that can be used to achieve specific goals:

- Education, training and development - providing these will ensure knowledge and skills are up to date and also instil confidence plus a motivation 'to want to change'.

- Coercion - threat of force. Often it is sufficient to use a tactic that proposes or implies a threat. This technique frequently results in individuals complying and modifying their behaviour.

Evaluating strategies and tactics

It is important that any strategy or tactic used is evaluated before being used again. Even though a tactic has not been effective in one situation it may be useful in another circumstance. The tendency to use the same set of tactics repeatedly without a 'built-in evaluation' should be avoided.

The same is true with matching strategies with tactics. If a strategy has been unsuccessful it does not necessarily mean the tactics selected and used need to be discarded. More importantly, when a new strategy is required the tactics should be selected as a 'new fit' to achieve the goals.

Summary

Change is constant. More than ever before, in a constantly changing National Health Service, midwifery managers and midwifery sisters must to be able to affect change quickly and efficiently, for continued success and survival in the internal market structure.

Change is often managed unsatisfactorily. People react to change in different ways and this is frequently ignored. Not all changes are resisted. Resistance to change can be good or bad. Negative resistance is more often due to the way the manager introduces a change than to the change itself.

Modern managers are now being encouraged to pay more attention to their organization's corporate culture, when carrying out change. This includes beliefs and values, norms and the style of management. Perception is formed by behaviour and the 'culture' of an organization can act as an accelerator or a brake as far as performance is concerned. Changing the organization's culture is a continuous process and will take time and energy. To do this midwifery managers must have a clear vision of what their Maternity Service wants to achieve for mothers and babies, and where it wants to be in the future. Essential is the commitment, acceptance and ownership of the change by the staff.

The process of change involves unfreezing, changing and refreezing. As each change-process is unique and each situation different, midwifery managers will need to work out various approaches, methods and strategies to achieve the desired goals

Force Field Analysis Theory is a useful planning tool to focus on the solution phase of problem solving, prior to changing a situation from actual to a desired optimal goal. By first identifying the Pushing and Restraining forces, change can be accomplished by augmenting the positive forces, or reducing the negative forces. The Conflict Theory in Change Management contends that most social changes are preceded by conflicting forces to prevent change. Strategies and tactics are necessary for planning and implementing change, especially with regard to *Changing Childbirth* (1993) and for overcoming what is described as 'normal' resistance.

CHAPTER FIVE

Managing Resources

'The enterprise, by definition, must be capable of producing more or better than all the resources that comprise it. It must be a genuine whole: greater than, or at least different from the sum of its parts, with its output larger than the sum of all its inputs' (Peter Drucker, 1979)

Over the last fifteen years the National Health Service has undergone a number of fundamental reforms which have had a major impact upon the way health services are provided. These include:

*   General management: The Griffiths Report (1983) led to the appointment of general managers in the NHS, a structure which has been strengthened in recent years. The intention of general management was to give responsibility to one person, at each level of the National Health Service, for planning, implementation, control of performance and continuous quality improvement in health care. General managers operate at district level, and in NHS Trusts.

*   Contractual funding: The separation of funding and provision, which was implemented as a result *Working for Patients* (1989) clarified the role of purchasers and providers of health care, and resulted in the 'Purchaser-Provider split'. The intention of contractual funding was to create competitiveness between providers of health care and improve quality of their services.

*   Resource management: This was an extension of the Griffiths Report (1983), which recommended doctors and nurses should take more control in the management of resources. The intention of resource management was to give doctors, midwives and nurses more accountability for the efficient and effective use of resources. This has led to the creation of Clinical Directorates in NHS Trusts, and the appointment of Clinical Directors.

Demands for an increase in resources for health care will always be infinite, but National Health Service funding is finite. Funding is a top-down approach, often based on mechanistic formulae, in an attempt to introduce objectivity and equity. Each year April to March, Health Authorities receive from the Department of Health a funding allocation, currently based on a 'capitation per head' formula for each member of the population in their geographical health district. General Practitioner (GP) fundholders will receive their budget allocation from this funding, for purchasing elective treatment and services on behalf of their patients. The major proportion of the funding will remain with the Health Authority, the main purchaser of health care for essential services such as maternity services, accident and emergency, medicine, care of the elderly and community services. Thus Health Authorities and GP fundholders purchase services through sound budgeting and contractual arrangements with NHS Trusts and other provider units, for example private hospitals, independent pathology services.

Against this background is the drive for economy, efficiency and effectiveness in the National Health Service with an emphasis on the reduction of waste, achievement of the best results from available resources and an increase in productivity. Fundamentally, lower costs and increased effectiveness are now the responsibility of NHS Trusts as the providers of services, but the momentum for the 'value for money' concept is still being driven by the Department of Health.

Many midwives and health professionals, on first impression, may find a concentration on economy, efficiency and value for money, an antithesis to their caring roles and the reasons why they chose to work in the National Health Service. With an understanding of the principles that govern the effective management of resources, it is anticipated that midwifery managers and midwives can be united in their efforts to provide Maternity Services that are efficient and meet the needs of mothers and babies. For the midwifery manager, one of the greatest challenges is human resource management. The *Changing Childbirth* report (1993) makes clear reference to midwives skills, that they should be fully utilized and reflect the full role for which the midwife has been trained. The rate of organizational change has never been greater, which means having people with the right skills capable of delivering strategies and achieving contracts. It is only through effective human resource management that these objectives can be met.

Understanding resources
Definitions
A resource is:

>'a means of satisfying a want or deficiency; capability in adapting means to ends or in meeting difficulties'.
>(Oxford English Dictionary)

>'source or possibility of help; an expedient; money or means of raising money'.
>(Chambers 20th Century Dictionary)

>'skill in devising means; means of supplying a want; stock that can be drawn on; means of support'.
>(Odhams Diamond Dictionary)

Categories of resources
There are two - primary and secondary.

- Primary - human resources which are divided into two groups: managers and workers

- Secondary - facilities (non human) which include money, materials, equipment, technology, motor vehicles, buildings, land.

Primary resources are the activators. They energize or convert the secondary resources to generate more resources. For example, midwives use a fetal monitor to check the fetal heart is within the normal range, in readiness for a natural confinement. Primary resources are the only resources capable of development and direct growth.

Secondary resources must be activated or converted before they can be used to generate more resources. For example, an unused fetal heart monitor is static, unproductive and ineffective.

Productivity

This is the efficiency of the activation or generation of resources. Productivity means the balance between all the factors of production which will give the greatest output for the least input. For example:

- by using the fetal heart monitor —> live healthy baby —> the midwife augments the quality of maternity care.

Not only is the midwife using the fetal heart monitor to ensure the birth of a live healthy baby but the parents are overjoyed with their baby's birth, which is good for the midwife, maternity service and the NHS Trust.

There is only one way secondary resources can grow and this is by the conversion of financial resources. For example: spending money to buy skilled midwives; purchasing computers and selling off second-hand equipment.

Secondary resources can grow indirectly, but can only do this as a result of the activities of primary resources.

In summary:
- primary resources are resource-users
- secondary resources are resource-convertors

The nature of primary resources

Managers
- are the activating agents of all other resources, both primary and secondary
- are a costly resource, but it is their efficiency in utilizing resources, converting and re-converting them to financial resources that is crucial to the NHS Trust.

Human beings
They have a set of qualities possessed by no other resources. The human resource has the ability to:

- coordinate
- integrate
- judge
- imagine.

Workers
They will determine:

- whether they will work at all
- how fast they will work
- the quality of their work - regardless of whether standards have been set and agreed
- whether to respond positively to external stimuli if they are appropriate or negatively to the same stimuli if they are not. Positive stimuli may be:
  - motivation
  - high morale
  - effective management
  - style of leadership
  - incentives and rewards
- whether they will generate resources at the same rate as that desired by management

Workers are generally gregarious and like to work in groups, which may be formal but are more likely to be informal. Both managers and workers can be developed in skills and attitudes.

The problems with primary resources
Although managers and workers can be educated and developed to become highly skilled practitioners and perform competently, the property in them does not belong to the Maternity Service or the NHS Trust.

Staff will remain in their jobs and with the NHS Trust only so long as:

- it suits them
- their loyalty remains to their formal groups - the organizational structure in which midwives work, and to informal groups - socializing with colleagues
- their satisfaction remains high e.g. pride in their job, their motivation and morale is upheld
- the pay and conditions are at least as good as anywhere else.

Therefore, the NHS Trust has a balance to keep. It must continue to recruit, appoint, and develop primary resources, and at the same time prepare to lose staff through retirement, resignations to work with another employer, transfer, sickness and death.

The nature of secondary resources

Assets

Secondary resources remain the property of the NHS Trust.

Money

Basically all business activities in the NHS Trust centre around the problems of using money for:

- services for customers, patients, mothers and babies
- paying staff - which accounts for around 80 per cent of total expenditure
- servicing equipment and buying new equipment.

Very minimal money is transmuted into yet more money.

Capacity

Secondary resources can only develop by increasing their uses up to maximum capacity e.g. utilization of clinic time and space.

The problems with secondary resources

Equipment depreciates and buildings require continuous maintenance to ensure they remain safe environments for patients, clients, visitors and staff. Problems arise when equipment wears out, needs repairing or replacing. Sometimes the original reasons for purchasing expensive equipment change, and alternative uses have to be developed.

Value for money

According to Perrin (1988), the 'Value for money' concept represents a concern of the government in that the National Health Service should be required to evaluate its own performance and should be audited and assessed independently to bring about improvements. This, Perrin says 'is all part of the present government's overall thrust to lower costs or improve performance'.

Achieving value for money is made up of two key stages:

- examining how the money is spent
- examining how the money might be spent more effectively.

When carrying out these examinations every aspect of the service has to be considered. For Maternity Services the following would need to be included:

- the way mothers and babies are actually cared for, and whether their needs are met
- the cost, standard and quality of the different types of care
- divisions of work between different types and grades of staff

- supplies, equipment and laundry etc.
- the systems for providing financial and clinical information.

Economy: efficiency and effectiveness

Statistics show that productivity in the National Health Service has increased during the last ten years. This is because the demand for health care and opportunities to provide this care have risen more rapidly than the funding and resources available. In consequence, resources in the National Health Service are 'tighter' than they have ever been. This means every possible assistance is required to achieve a better understanding of resources, their management and control.

Providing financial and workload information will help midwifery managers, clinicians, midwives and staff to understand how to achieve the best maternity services 'outputs' for mothers and babies from limited resources. Financial and workload information can provide:

- detailed documentational evidence of sound resource management
- accurate information when 'putting in a bid' for an increase in resource allocation.

In practical terms, to understand economy, efficiency and effectiveness it is first necessary to have an awareness of inputs, outputs and outcomes.

Inputs

These are the resources that are used to obtain something, provide something or get something done. These include primary resources (managers and workers) and secondary resources (equipment, buildings, energy sources and money in order to purchase other resources).

Outputs

These are the number of things or activities that are provided or get done. These include:

- number of mothers delivered
- number of babies born
- number of miles travelled
- number of packs used.

Outcomes

These give the quality in outputs and are usually the most difficult to define, measure and cost. These include:

- meeting the needs of each mother and baby through successful management of their maternity care
- successful interventions and treatments in maternity care
- satisfaction levels of mothers

Costs of inputs have always been recorded and monitored, but now there is a requirement to record the exact use, or the consumption of input-resources when producing outputs. This information can be obtained by measuring:

- activity
- workload
- throughput
- monitoring performance.

Some outputs can be classified as 'intermediate'. For example, the use of the ultrasound scan is a means to achieving a preferred final output and outcome in childbirth. In other words, the scan is used to exclude fetal abnormality and therefore contributes to the birth of a healthy newborn baby.

Understanding economy: efficiency and effectiveness

Perrin (1988) calls these the 'three Es'. Each one has an important role in the management of National Health Services resources. Unfortunately, as he says, the use of the words economy, efficiency and effectiveness cause many health professionals to instinctively react against such concepts, believing they are the opposite to their caring roles. Nevertheless, the 'three Es' are significant in practical terms to ensure the best possible use of resources in the care of mothers and babies.

ECONOMY

This simply means avoiding waste:
- it is an uncomplicated concept because it does not consider the outputs accomplished in using resources
- means spending and consuming as little as possible. For example, electricity, swabs, paper-towels, envelopes etc.
- is expressed in basic cost figures, and recorded. For example, miles per gallon, cost per ultrasound scan, cost per meal etc.
- on its own it has limited application to managers, but can be used to encourage staff to be more economical. For example: by switching lights off in the daylight; taking the shortest route by road when visiting a mother in her own home.

EFFICIENCY

This is a more complex concept:
- it takes into account the output as well as the input
- is expressed as a direct or joined relationship between the output and input
- becomes a useful measure when connected to other factors. For example, miles per gallon is meaningless on its own, but when related to the number of home visits by a community midwife it becomes meaningful. Cost per ultrasound becomes significant when related to antenatal screening and the reduction of babies born with fetal congenital abnormalities
- can be improved by either increasing the output but maintaining or reducing the input or keeping the output the same but reducing the input

- is about controlling. Unnecessary tests, i.e. routine Hb tests in the early postnatal period, empty beds, unused rooms in antenatal clinics so that resources can be spread across the Maternity Services for improvements.

EFFECTIVENESS

This is a refined concept relating to the volume and cost of outputs and the quality achieved in outcomes. It:

- suggests a benefit is achieved from the use of resources in one activity as compared with another
- includes 'Opportunity Costs' - An 'Opportunity Cost' is a chance to use resources from one activity to another which might have a higher value or benefit. For example, the opportunity to amalgamate two antenatal Parent Education courses into one course for six months is made possible due to a reduction in mothers booking for antenatal care. This enables a midwife to be released to commence a much needed 'Pre Conception Clinic' for teenagers.
- incorporates 'maternity care outcomes' - which provide information on the state of the health and wellbeing of mothers and babies. The problem is that not many systems are available to measure in terms of objectivity and that will allow judgements to be made between comparative benefits and effectiveness. For example, when a decision has been made to shift more resources for antenatal screening tests and less for neonatal intensive care.
- is a means of monitoring quality (as far as is measurable) and assessing whether the needs of consumers are met. In practice the use of the word 'effectiveness' is often reduced to mean the same as 'efficiency'. For example, when resources are expressed in financial terms, the measure then becomes a cost effectiveness indicator.

Resource management

The idea for resource management originated from the *Griffiths Inquiry* into NHS Management (1983). In this report Griffiths argued that hospital doctors should accept responsibility for management.

The Resource Management Iniative (RMI) commenced in 1987. The key aim as stated by the NHS Management Executive (August, 1987) was for the NHS 'to give a better service to patients by helping clinicians and other managers to make more informed judgements about how the resources they control can be used to maximum effect'. Six 'Acute Hospital' pilot sites were set up during 1987 and 1988 to test the concept of clinical management in practice, and each reported back favourably. Twenty more hospital units were then identified to follow these, and through a phase-in programme resource management has gradually been implemented.

Although the aim of the Resource Management Iniative was to bring direct management to 'clinicians', meaning doctors, midwives, nurses and other professional clinical staff, there is no doubt that the main target was the doctors. In managers eyes doctors were an elite group of professionals who possessed in depth scientific knowledge and held extraordinary power within the National Health Service. Midwives and nurses in contrast, as observed by Robinson and Strong (1992) represented collective feebleness, who were weak in influence, and in professions where there was little scientific base.

Directorate management structures

The basic model for Resource management is the triangular structure (Fig.5.1) where the Clinical Director (sometimes known as Clinical Co-ordinator) has managerial responsibility for the budget, clinical activity and the operational performance of all the staff in the directorate, and is typically assisted by a midwifery or nurse manager and by a business manager. Recently, there has been a move away from this model, mainly because of the unclear demarcation between the two manager roles which frequently resulted in duplication of effort. In its place the duumvirate structure has emerged (Fig. 5.2), with a clinical director and a service or directorate manager. The service manager being a combination of the midwifery or nurse manager role and that of the business manager. This move has led to mainly previous business managers being appointed to these posts, and consequently midwifery and nurse managers have been lost through early retirement or redundancy.

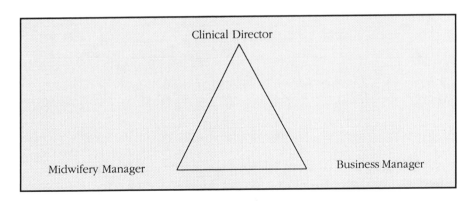

Fig. 5.1: The traditional Clinical Directorate structure

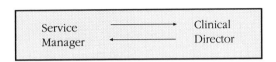

Fig. 5.2: The new duumvirate system for Clinical Directorate Management

An alternative model, which recognizes the professional and clinical role of the managers, is one based on the 'Knowhow Organization' of Sveiby and Bloomsbury (Fig. 5.3). This thrives on variety and adaptability and is different from a NHS Trust that operates a service which emphasizes standardization, consistency and continuity and where the centre is in control. NHS Trusts that have implemented clinical directorate systems already recognize the emphasis placed on devolution, by giving responsibility to those at the level where clinical care is provided and involving clinicians in management. For effective management of clinical directorates, this requires a high level of professional and management 'knowhow', which needs to be balanced. Therefore management is best in the 'hands' of those professionals who can manage and deliver health care. For example, the medical and midwifery professionals with additional management and business skills.

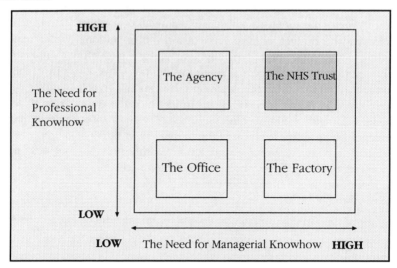

Fig. 5.3: Showing the requirement for balance of high managerial and professional knowhow in the NHS Trust

Regardless of the directorate structure chosen, Spurgeon (1993) points out there is still much work to be done in developing the management skills of Clinical Directors. The majority of these posts have been filled by consultants who have come from a self-contained medical culture to one of collective decision-making about health care, and priorities and options. As for clinical midwifery managers they may find themselves in the centre, responsible managerally to the Clinical Director, professionally to the NHS Director of Nursing and Midwifery, but reporting on a daily basis to the service manager.

Clinical Resource Management involves:

• clinicians being included in management decisions.
• delegation of day to day management responsibilities to clinical teams, giving them more accountability for decision-making and the quality aspects of health care.
• using fully integrated information systems to support clinical, operational and management functions and decision-making.
• providing the opportunity for greater efficiency whereby releasing more resources for direct clinical care.
• clinical and medical audit leading to improved agreed standards of health care.
• more responsive management which is closer to the level of clinical care and service provision.

The benefits are:

- resource management has enabled managers and clinicians to come together and consider directly what are the costs of various types of health care, to contemplate alternatives and make decisions in a more informed way.
- decision-making is made at the level where clinical care and services are provided.
- through information technology systems links can be made between clinical activity data, resource allocations and costs.

Managing human resources

'People are our most important asset' is a saying frequently quoted by managers everywhere, and yet according to Pearson and Thomas (1991) in many organizations people remain under-valued, under-trained and under-utilized.

For NHS Trusts and maternity services to survive and prosper into the 21st Century there is no doubt more radical approaches to managing people will need to be considered and practised. The impact of medical and obstetric advances, the accelerating use of technology, increased consumer expectations and the purchaser-provider split mean NHS Trusts as employers will have to be more flexible and responsive than they have in the past. The rate of change has never been greater than it is now, which means Trusts will need to employ the right people with the right skills, capable of delivering the Trust's strategies and meeting the needs of consumers.

People as assets to an organization is an interesting concept. Handy (1993) accepts it is fashionable to talk about human assets, but also believes that in doing so this acts as a reminder that human resources need 'maintenance and proper utilization', to ensure their outputs are greater than their costs. He even goes as far as suggesting that perhaps one day administrative organizations will start behaving like 'football clubs where players are truthfully human assets', and charge realistic transfer fees for their key people-assets. The care and protection given to key assets by leading 'football clubs' is one where training and development become vital, increasing their productive potential and leading to greater efficiency. In this way the asset becomes appreciated in terms of capital value.

Despite the generally accepted view that human resources are valuable, the drive for more economy, efficiency and effectiveness in the National Health Service has led to the current debate as to how human resources should be managed. Flanagan (1993) asserts this has engendered a climate of cost-minimization and caused senior health service managers to reduce the cost of labour and deal with people as 'factors of production'. The debate centres on whether to develop a 'hard' or 'soft' approach to managing human resources. The 'hard' focuses on the resource itself, whereas the 'soft' concentrates on the human side of the resource.

Hard

The human resource is no different from any other resource:

- people are there to be managed
- purchased as cheaply as possible
- developed and exploited as fully and profitable as possible
- is supportive of sub-contracting
- is about making the corporate business work.

Soft

Focuses on the human side:

- although people are usually a most expensive resource they are crucial for turning other resources into valuable outputs
- people can be creative and commit themselves
- people skills can generate a real 'competitive edge' to standards and quality of care
- people require careful selection, nurturing, proper rewards and integration into the organization.

Needless to say the 'soft' approach is the one that has been formally adopted by most NHS Trusts. It remains to be seen whether the pressure on Trusts to perform effectively and competitively and to keep within budget, will force them to accept in part elements of a more hard approach.

Human Resource Management

Human Resource Management (HRM) is different from the traditional personnel management function. HRM is principally concerned with organizing staff in such a way that is beneficial in achieving the NHS Trust's purpose, whereas personnel management is an attempt to bring about productivity in a more systematic way within the Trust's business plan.

HRM starts from the time a NHS Trust requires human resources to convert secondary resources into productivity for the benefit of people using the health service. The focus is on demand rather than supply, on direction rather than problem-solving and by developing strategies to meet the needs of the NHS Trust. The essential requirement is employee cooperation, and this can be achieved by creating the right corporate culture, and through remuneration packages, teamworking and management development. Flanagan (1993) believes it is 'the goal of commitment, where employees have a much closer identity with the organization's growth and prosperity', that separates human resource management from personnel management. Staff become committed rather than simply following agreed procedures.

Human resource strategies have been developed in NHS Trusts and as a result three similar patterns have been seen to emerge:

- a close integration between human resource management, the corporate culture and the business strategy

- a more independent approach to employment practices, including pay policies, conditions of service, remuneration packages and minimal influence by trade unions.

- a preference to select and recruit as the Trust considers necessary, by limiting and controlling employment contracts i.e. short term contracts, and concentrating on training and development.

The success of a human resource strategy in practice is dependent on all those in management positions, and cannot be left to just a few senior managers. Midwifery managers and midwifery sisters will be required to manage people in the most effective way, through leadership, motivation, development and empowering staff. As Drummond (1991) says the ideal state to aim for is where the job virtually becomes a hobby. One where there is obvious enjoyment and where people can shine through. This may be utopia, but its well worth aiming for!

The human resource strategy

Human resourcing is about:

- selecting }
- rewarding }   people to enable the NHS Trust to achieve its goals.
- developing }

In the same way that the NHS Trust requires strategies for business, marketing and information technology, it also requires a 'people' strategy. In developing a human resources strategy there are two main questions to be asked:

- what type of staff are needed to meet the Trust's strategic objectives i.e. providing treatments and care in the range of 'health specialities' supplied and meeting the needs of consumers.

- what people systems must be designed and implemented to develop and retain staff with the appropriate skills and who practice competently and effectively.

A NHS Trust without a human resources strategy is at risk of becoming vulnerable to external factors. In the present climate of the internal market external factors could easily dominate the way the Trust operates, and even dictate its future direction. With a human resources strategy the Trust is able to plan effectively for its people and services, to drive its own course of action and control its future. Because of uncertainty about future contracts, possible reductions in funding and the need to rationalize services, the strategy must reflect the real situation in the workplace. Usually the strategy covers a five year period, but because of the many uncertainties an update annually will ensure it reflects what is actually happening. Figure 5.4 shows how the Human Resources Strategy relates to other key aspects of the NHS Trust.

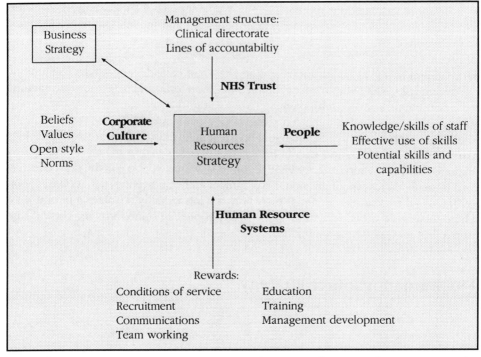

Fig. 5.4: Showing how the human resources strategy relates to other systems in the NHS Trusts (adapted from Pearson and Thomas, 1991).

The human resource strategy usually includes:

Finding out exactly the present and required abilities of staff

The absolute aim being to plan the match of demand and supply, and to ensure there is no excess waste in the number of staff and their skills. By assessing what knowledge, skills and experience people currently have, and what they require in order to meet the changing needs of the service, the NHS Trust can plan effectively in utilizing skills and meeting the changing needs of the service (Fig. 5.5).

Establishing external human resource trends

This is usually achieved by working closely with outside agencies, i.e. the NHS Training Directorate, Universities and merged Colleges of Nursing and Midwifery, and other agencies to ensure the NHS Trust is up-to-date with trends in human resourcing, health care practices and developments.

Linking the human resource strategy to the business strategy

The business of the NHS Trust can only be achieved when staff have the right knowledge and skills, are properly trained and developed, and the skills are used effectively in the right circumstances and for the right people.

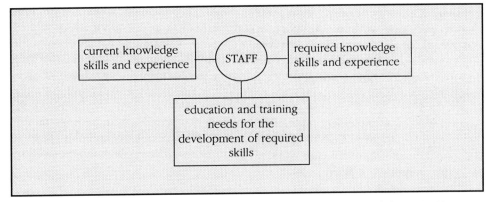

Fig. 5.5: Asssssing the requirements to meet the changing needs of the NHS Trust

Employee relations
This includes the local negotiation of pay and terms and conditions of service with representatives of the Professional Associations and Trade Unions and through grading and job evaluation, industrial relations, grievance, discipline and employment legislation.

Employee resources
This includes manpower planning, recruitment and selection, equal opportunities, skill-mix, sickness and absenteeism, training of health care assistants, flexible working arrangements, individual and team reward, performance agreements, financial rewards and 'Opportunity 200' which particularly promotes sexual equality in jobs.

Employee development
This includes individual performance review, management development, post basic education and training, non-clinical training, career development and succession planning.

Skill mix
Skill mix is achieving the right balance between qualified and unqualified staff, and trained and untrained staff. It involves identifying the range of practices, responsibilities and tasks involved in providing care e.g. for Maternity Services, the level of skills required and who should carry them out. When future needs are different to those currently being provided it may be necessary for staff to attain new skills, or for the midwifery manager to change the balance of trained to untrained staff, or to increase or reduce the numbers of staff in post. Skill mix studies have shown that people in higher graded posts e.g. managers and sisters are often the ones who undertake junior skills and lower skilled duties.

The ideal skill mix is achieved when the level of service is provided and the standards of care are met within the finance available. It ensures the best possible use of scarce professional skills to maximize the quality of health care.

Job sharing is a way of opening up posts that have only been available on a full time basis to part time workers. In theory, according to Walton (1990) all jobs could be considered for job share, which involves two people sharing one full time post, and dividing the salary, holidays and other benefits between them. It is a way of improving the quality of part time work and increasing the access to higher graded midwifery posts.

Support workers complement professional midwifery practitioners and are essential to the work of midwives. Due to changes in midwifery education and the move to vocational qualifications for care workers, the nursing auxiliary has been replaced by two new categories of health workers:

- the maternity care assistant - usually appointed following a skill mix review. Pay and conditions being determined locally.

- the maternity care support worker - who holds a vocational qualification and provides support to the professional work of the midwife. She or he who will work under the direction of the midwife who remains accountable for appropriate delegation and supervision of the work done.

Communications

These recognize the importance of effective communication with and between staff, and develop ways of achieving sound communications processes and practices. This involves creating an 'open' communication culture, which includes every member of staff.

Patients Charter

This includes the setting and agreeing of standards with staff, and monitoring their effectiveness in the clinical environment to ensure a high quality service is provided.

Health at work

Meeting the objectives that are specified in the governments 'Health at Work Iniative', including policies for healthy eating; developing a smoke free environment and alcohol at work.

Customer relations

The provision of training for staff in customer awareness, consumer feedback and how to ensure a quality health service.

EEC legislation

Managers and staff must ensure that they work within the legal framework of the single European market, changing their working practices as necessary. The main changes are those that affect the Health and Safety of employees, especially with regard to pregnant staff.

Reward packages

These are essential to the success of the NHS Trust. It is a requirement to ensure staff have job satisfaction, feel valued and fit into the corporate culture. Although financial rewards are a significant part of work other factors are equally important. Flexible reward packages can provide a further dimension to employment and increase motivation at work. These include job share, flexible working arrangements, home working, term-time working, benefit packages, career breaks, annual hours contracts and pre-retirement schemes.

Recruitment and selection of staff

Recruitment is one of the biggest challenges for midwifery managers in the 1990s. The purpose of recruitment and selection is to match the characteristics of individuals - their skills, knowledge and interests - to the current and anticipated demands for jobs. Having the right staff with the right skills will be necessary to implement the recommendations of *Changing Childbirth* (1993).

New methods of recruitment will be required, along with tried-and tested traditional methods, as will innovative flexible working arrangements.

Determining a vacancy

Potential vacancies occur when a midwife or maternity support worker decides to leave her job or a new post is created as a result of expansion. There are two questions the midwifery manager must answer:

- is there a vacancy?
- is the vacancy to be filled by another person?

Recruiting another person into the post may seem the most obvious, but before doing this automatically the midwifery manager will need to consider whether there are any other ways of fulfilling the work in this post:

- Can the work be reorganized? Hints that this may be a possibility may be obtained during the 'pre-leaving' interview with the previous post holder. If the reason a secretary gives for leaving is because of insufficient work to do, or a midwife says the established team workers in a ward have not been receptive to her in her job, then reorganizing the work may be an option. Also, if work in another area of the Maternity Services is being reduced, midwives and staff can be redeployed.

- Can the post be made part time or one that can be achieved by flexible working hours? Torrington and Hall (1991) tell us that replacing full time jobs with part time jobs has the attraction of making marginal reductions more possible and at the same time provides the possibility of marginally increasing the amount of staff time available by redefining the job as full time.

- Would it be better to use the midwives bank? - Temporary and casual staff allow for flexibility and at the same time provide space for job reassessment. In a climate of competitiveness, short contracts, rationalization and streamlining bank midwives see themselves as marketable and have much to offer in terms of skills, interest and commitment. It is important, however, that prior to appointing a midwife to the bank proper interview and selection techniques are used.

- What about using nursing agencies or sub-contracting the work? These are ways of avoiding ongoing costs and obligations for the NHS Trust by transferring these to another employer.

When a decision is made to recruit into the vacant post the following issues will need to be assessed:

- what will the post consist of?
- will the post be any different from that carried out by the previous post-holder?
- will the post be suitable for a job share?
- will the job description need updating or rewriting?
- what aspects of the post will specify the type of person suitable for the post?
- what is to be included in the 'Person Specification'?
- which key aspects of the post are to be used for advertising and recruitment purposes?

Recruitment methods

It is important to choose the method which is most appropriate for midwifery recruitment and one that is cost effective. There are numerous methods to choose from which include:

- Internal advertising:
  - Notice boards
  - Recruitment bulletins
- Advertisements in:
  - Local press
  - Midwifery and nursing press
  - National press
- Job centres
- Midwifery and nursing agencies
- Recruitment and search consultants
- Career conventions
- Open days
- Radio advertising

Writing the advertisement

Deciding what to include in the advertisement is important because of the need to:

- attract the attention of the right people
- keep costs to a minimal

Usually the use of key words will achieve both these objectives.

The following points also need to be included in the advert:
- the name of the NHS Trust and the specific name of the Maternity Services Unit
- the title of the post and a few of the main duties
- the key points of the 'person specification' i.e. qualifications, previous experience etc.
- grade of post and salary
- how to find out more information about the post e.g. by telephoning, by informal discussion, by writing for details
- how to apply - by application form or CV or both - and where to send the application
- closing date for applications and date of interview.

The recruitment process

From the start of the recruitment process the midwifery manager will need to work closely with the Clinical Director, the personnel or human resources manager and the recruitment office.

The following documentation will need to be prepared and available for interested applicants and is usually presented in an 'information pack'.

- Job description
- Person specification
- Literature about the Maternity Services, the NHS Trust and other local interests
- Equal opportunities form
- Application form
- Health declaration form and a pre-addressed envelope to the Occupational Health Department for returning the completed form.

The documentation required for the recruitment process and monitoring purposes is as follows:

- Copy of the advertisement
- A system for recording the names, addresses and other details of interested people and applicants.
- Standard letters of correspondence to be sent with the information pack and following short-listing
- Miscellaneous information - notifying telephonists about general enquiries, informing receptionists about pending visits of interested persons to the Maternity Unit and the candidates for interview

Shortlisting

It is essential that shortlisting is fair and objective. This is best carried out by the members of the intended interview panel, or at least two members of the panel. The benefits of careful shortlisting are:

- it increases the fairness to all candidates and removes bias
- it reduces the chance of calling unsuitable candidates for interview
- it provides the interview panel with an opportunity of working together and clarifying goals.

The numerical method of shortlisting is considered to be the fairest for objectivity. This can be carried out using the following process:

- agree the essential criteria for shortlisting
- agree the number of candidates to be called for interview
- enter the agreed criteria onto the shortlisting grid (Fig. 5.6)

Essential Criteria Marked out of ten (10)	Candidate Number						
	1	2	3	4	5	6	7
Qualifications: Registered Midwife Diploma or degree in Midwifery							
Experience: Ward/departmental management Team midwifery, mentor to students							
Practical and Intellectual skills: Range of clinical skills, leadership and communication skills							
Continuing/inservice education: Recent attendance at study days, reference to 'Changing Childbirth'							
Personal circumstances: Car driver, clean licence, lives within 10 miles of maternity unit							
Total marks							
Ranking order							

Name of assessor ———— Signature of assessor ———— Date of shortlisting

Fig. 5.6: Shortlisting grid giving examples of 'essential criteria' for a midwife's post

- give each candidate a number and enter that number on:
  - the corner of their application form and CV
- each member of the shortlisting panel will asses each candidate:
  - by using the agreed criteria and giving a numerical award for each criteria based on information provided by the candidate
  - by adding up the numerical awards and giving a total for each candidate.

From comparing the 'totals' the candidates will be put in priority order i.e. the highest score will be candidate number one, the lowest score will be the last candidate

- the shortlisting panel now come together and share their priority order findings. These are added together (Fig. 5.7) and now the lowest scores will determine which candidates will be called for interview.

Candidate Number	Three shortlisting assessors Ranking order of each	Total	Final ranking order (of total)	Candidate invited for interview
1	5 : 3 : 2	10	3	✓
2	1 : 2 : 1	4	1	✓
3	2 : 1 : 3	6	2	✓
4	3 : 6 : 5	14	5	–
5	4 : 5 : 4	13	4	–
6	6 : 4 : 6	16	16	–

Fig. 5.7: Showing how three candidates are selected for interview using shortlisting grid

Methods of selection

Selection is important for ensuring, as far as possible, which applicants will be the most suitable for accomplishing the requirements of the job. Significantly there are costs associated with poor selection. If the wrong appointment is made this can bring with it a whole series of problems, and could mean the person appointed is with the Maternity Services for a long time.

Today selection is a two way process. At various stages decisions will be made by the midwifery manager acting as the employer, and by the potential employee - the applicant. Throughout the selection process applicants can choose whether to proceed or not, based on the way they perceive the information is given, their assessment of the informal discussion and whether they are offered another post. This perspective is the opposite to the traditional view of employment, which supports a management led approach for selection and appointment. Midwifery managers need to accept that they do not have total control over who is appointed because of this two-way system that now operates. Sometimes the best candidates withdraw, leaving unsuitable applicants. In these circumstances it is far better to readvertise than to appoint the wrong person for the sake of haste.

Application form

This usually provides personal information; a synopsis of the applicant's professional qualifications and work history. Application forms provide essential information for shortlisting, for preparing for the interview and during the interview itself.

Curriculum Vitae (CV)

This is a previously prepared personal profile and professional history, which is becoming more popular in an age of word processors and computers. However, it is more subject to manipulation than an application form; the latter more often being completed in the candidate's own handwriting. There is, however, a place for both methods.

Telephone screening

If speed is important prospective candidates can be selected and interview dates arranged over the phone. For this method to be effective a checklist of crucial questions has to be prepared in advance. Each telephone candidate is asked the same questions, and from their responses selection is made to attend for interview. However, the midwifery manager needs to use this method with caution because:

- of the difficulty with setting standard questions in advance
- there is no time for reflection prior to offering a date for interview
- as enquiries continue to come in there may be a realization that the best candidates phoned in early but because standards were originally set high they were not asked to attend for interview.

Testing

The use of tests in appointment procedures is full of arguments for and against. Those who support testing do so because they believe the interview alone is not reliable. Jordan (1987) points to evidence of profound and fundamental biases which invade our assessments of others. Supporters assert the tests lead to greater objectivity and accuracy, and give credibility to decisions concerning selection. Those against, do not accept the objectivity of testing and find difficulty in accepting the evidence as part of the overall selection process.

APTITUDE TESTS

These measure a person's potential to develop in a specific or general way. When assessing the results it does not necessarily mean that a high level of aptitude converts into a high level of performance in a certain job. What it does indicate is that there is potential, but other factors such as motivation and ability also have to be considered for a high level of performance in a post.

PERSONALITY TESTS

Personality is difficult to measure. Not only because personality itself has many definitions but because, as Torrington and Hall (1991) say, it is dangerous to assume there is a standard profile of an ideal employee. Another difficulty is that the tests rely on a person's honesty. If performance tests are used there must be qualified personnel available to carry out the assessments.

Formal presentation

The practice of inviting candidates to give a short prepared presentation during interview is becoming popular. Generally the subject is chosen by the interview panel following shortlisting, and this will usually reflect issues directly associated with the post. Candidates are informed about the presentation at the same time as they are invited to the interview. The presentation will usually last between ten and fifteen minutes, dependent on the subject and the seniority of the post.

The formal presentation gives each candidate an opportunity to
- undertake preparatory work through research
- plan and write a structured presentation
- show an understanding of the subject and its association to the post
- choose which presentation-aids to use
- demonstrate their delivery and presentation skills.

There are also advantages for the interview panel. Presentations serve as a focus for:
- evaluating a candidate's knowledge and understanding of a subject
- assessing their motivation, clarity of delivery and presentation skills
- providing a forum for formulating specific questions, and evaluating the candidate's ability to answer clearly
- comparing candidates with one another.

However, caution needs to be exercised. For some candidates merely the suggestion of giving a presentation is sufficient to make them withdraw from an interview. On balance, presentations are more suitable for senior staff interviews, such as midwifery managers and midwifery sisters. This is because there is an expectation that those holding management posts would be able to conceptualize, communicate effectively and have clear presentation skills.

The selection interview

The purposes of the selection interview are:

- to obtain information from a person, by assessing their responses against pre-selected criteria, and forecasting how successfully they will perform in the post for which they are applying
- to give the candidate details about the post and the organization to facilitate them with their decision as to whether they would accept the post.

During an interview the conversation is controlled, and there will be a higher rate of exchange in a much shorter period than in ordinary conversation.

Preparing for the interview

SELECTION OF THE INTERVIEW PANEL

Panel interviewing demonstrates fairness, and according to Muir (Torrington and Hall, 1991) it is less influenced by personal bias. Panel interviews also allow the candidate to get a better feel of the organization. When deciding how many interviewers to have, three or four is a suitable number for a professional midwifery interview. More than four could be intimidating for the candidate. Two or less could lead to bias. A suggested composition for an interview panel to appoint a midwifery sister is:

- Clinical Director
- midwifery manager
- personnel manager or representative
- outside assessor: midwifery manager or educationalist.

A suggested composition for an interview panel to appoint a midwife is:

- midwifery manager
- personnel manager or representative
- midwifery sister
- outside assessor: midwifery manager; educationalist or sister.

INTERVIEW BRIEFING

Each interviewer will require the following:

* copies of the job description and person specification
* a copy of each completed application form and CV
* charts and records for preparing their own notes and questions
* to meet together prior to the interview to agree the format of the interview and to clarify any points regarding the candidates.

TIMING OF INTERVIEWS

The time allocated for each candidate must be planned in advance. It is important that timing is realistic, e.g. if forty five minutes is considered ideal for each interview - allow one hour. This will ensure each interview starts on time, and will permit for the update of notes. A rigid timetable can cause too much strain on both sides, and can lead to frustrations and disappointments. A candidate still waiting long after her appointment time may become anxious and frustrated and this could jeopardise her performance during interview. Also it could give out the wrong signals about the Maternity Services and the NHS Trust.

RECEPTION

Clear written instructions should be sent to each candidate regarding the location of the interview and where to report. Reception staff must be informed when to expect candidates and their names, and what directions to give to the candidates e.g. whether someone will accompany them to the interview venue or alternatively where to direct the candidate.

VENUE FOR INTERVIEWS

The interview room should allow for private conversation, be free from interruptions and intrusions, and if possible away from noise. The room needs to be light and airy; not too big which gives a feeling of emptiness, and not too small so everyone feels cramped. The layout of the room is important and should encourage naturalness, so that candidates do not feel threatened. In this way they will be more forthcoming with information. Two types of layouts are usually preferred:

1. The open circular style (Fig. 5.8)

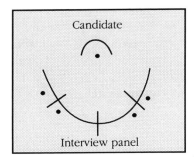

Fig. 5.8: Open circular style of interviewing

Advantages
•   there are no barriers
•   communication is direct and open

Disadvantages
•   the candidate may feel exposed
•   there is nowhere for interviewers and candidates to put their forms, papers etc.

2. Behind a desk or table (Fig. 5.9)

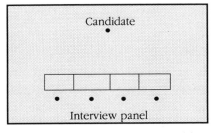

Fig. 5.9: Behind a desk or table

Advantage
- somewhere to put forms, papers etc.

Disadvantages
- acts as a barrier to communication
- distances the interviewers from the candidate

A good compromise can be attained by providing side desks or tables whist retaining the circular structure (Fig. 5.10).

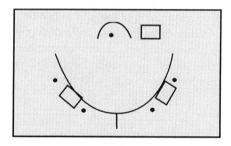

Fig. 5.10: Showing the circular layout with small tables for papers and forms

Conducting the interview

The interview needs to be structured because:

- candidates expect this
- it is professional
- it will help to ensure everything is covered for each candidate
- it aids memory recall for the interviewers and facilitates making notes immediately after the interview of each candidate
- it facilitates the comparison of candidates for decision-making.

The midwifery manager will usually chair the interviews for midwifery appointments and will oversee that each interview is structured and systematically worked through. The structure of an interview has the following pattern.

BEGINNING
This is when the candidate is greeted, introduced to the panel and put at ease. The chairperson will then briefly go through the application form, CV, clarify any points and ask for additional information e.g. anything that has been omitted from the application form.

MIDDLE
This section allows for discussion to take place by asking the candidate questions and listening to answers, obtaining information and maintaining rapport. This can be done through each interviewer asking questions in turn and the candidate also being invited to ask questions.

END
Bringing the interview to a close. The chairperson checks the candidate has no more questions, summarizes and indicates what will happen next e.g. when the result of the interview will be notified.

The interview process

Interviewers will be required to:

- Observe the candidate's manner: whether at ease or tense, appearance and dress, the tone of voice and the way questions are responded to.

- Keep questions clear and not too lengthy: Using open questions is best. Those beginning with 'w' will get more information. e.g. 'When did you...' 'What prompted you...' 'Where were you...' Closed questions are good for clarifying but should otherwise be discouraged.

  Listen not only to the answers to questions but to changes in tone and the pace of the reply. This will provide the interviewer with an opportunity to ask more questions and pursue a subject further.

The style and the personality of the interviewer can assist the candidate to be at ease:

- Showing interest, acknowledging a response, smiling and eye to eye contact all show sensitive awareness.

- Making notes - records are important, although some interviewers seem reluctant to make them. Notes can be made on the application form in advance of the interview, and the use of an 'interview plan' is recommended (Fig. 5.11)

Name of Candidate _____	Post _____	Date of interview _____
Outline of Question	Response of Candidate	Interviewer's Remarks
Name of interviewer _____	Signature of interviewer _____	

Figure 5.11: Interview question plan

The advantages of using an interview plan are:

* it allows questions to be written in advance, based on information in the application form and CV, the job description and person specification
* it provides a place for recording a summary of the candidate's response
* it provides a place for making additional remarks
* it is a permanent record for filing purposes.

Checking certificates

These include: birth certificate, certificates pertaining to educational and professional qualifications and evidence of further education and training. Before appointing a midwife it is essential that her registration is verified with the UKCC for Nursing, Midwifery and Health Visiting. This can be achieved by telephoning the UKCC on a specially agreed number for the NHS Trust.

Health clearance

Before a candidate is offered a post she will have to undergo health checks and be cleared by the Occupational Health Department as fit for employment. In the wake of the Beverley Allitt case, the *Clothier Enquiry* Report (1994) recommends that Occupational Health Departments should have access to sickness records from any institution an applicant has attended or been employed by. Also candidates with major personality disorders should be barred from the nursing and midwifery professions.

References

Candidates are usually asked to give the names of two referees, one of which is the present or previous employer. In practice the use of references is fraught with difficulties. Candidates are unlikely to give the name of a referee who will indicate they are unsuitable for the job, and that is why the employment reference is asked for. However, this is still problematic because some employers lack awareness about the job being applied for. Others may intentionally mislead by giving a glowing reference about a person they wish to lose or an unfavourable reference about a person they wish to retain. It is best to leave written references unread until after the interviews, and to read only when decisions have been made as to the selected candidate. In this way bias is avoided before the interview, all the interviewers have the opportunity to read the references at the same time, and references can be used as a backup to decisions already made. The use of telephone references is becoming much more widespread. Advocates of this argue it is fairer, it is more spontaneous therefore making it difficult for the referee to mislead, and of course questions can be asked and answers clarified.

Selecting the right candidate

Judgement should wait until after all the interviews have been completed. Selecting the right candidate will depend on:

- matching the person to the demands of the post
- matching the person to the culture of the Maternity Services and the NHS Trust
- comparing each candidate with the other candidates.

Selection is usually carried out by:

- sharing information and the assessments of each candidate
- asking each interviewer to briefly give their comments and assessment of each candidate so that a candidate is discussed one at a time. This includes:
  - assessing the actual responses to questions
  - the way the candidate responded
  - motivational factors
  - special aptitudes revealed
  - previous attainments
  - any prejudices disclosed
- coming to a census agreement as to which candidate is the most suitable and should be offered the post.

Although selection is subjective and often accompanied by elements of intuition, it does allow for comparative judgement and decision-making. More objective methods have been tried, using a points system, but many people are concerned that the element of human judgement is too closely proscribed.

Offer to selected candidate
This can be accomplished either by:

- telephone - with a follow-up letter confirming the offer
- letter offering the post.

Before contacting the selected candidate the panel needs to decide what to do in the event of the first choice turning down the job offer. Is there a second choice, or are there no other candidates suitable for the post?

In accepting the post the selected candidate will be required to confirm acceptance of the position in writing. Once this has been received, a letter of appointment can be sent by the midwifery manager or the personnel department. This will include:

- the date of commencement
- confirmation of grade and salary
- a brief summary of the terms and conditions of service.

An induction or orientation programme will need to be planned for the new midwife or a new member of staff. This will be tailored to any specific personal requirements (established during the interview), the needs of the job and the needs of the service. The programme should be sent to the midwife prior to the commencement date, and to each of the people and clinical areas involved in the induction.

The advantages of an induction programme for midwives are:

- it focuses on the new midwife - on her needs and what she should know
- it provides the new midwife with an opportunity to meet senior managers, colleagues and other professionals who she may not otherwise come into direct contact with on a daily basis
- it helps established midwives to remember what it was like to be new, and how best to help their new colleague
- it provides detailed information about the Maternity Services, its structure, policies and practices, in a relatively short period of time.
- it prepares the new midwife to take on her new role.

Post interview counselling for unsuccessful candidates

Unsuccessful candidates should be offered post interview counselling, which is usually given by the outside assessor. This can be given over the telephone or during face to face discussion. The method is agreed according to the candidates wishes, and the availability and accessibility of the assessor. The advantages of post interview counselling are:

- it gives the candidate opportunity to reflect on their performance during interview
- it provides a forum for open discussion about how the candidate performed
- the assessor can give advice to help the candidate with future applications
- it gives a positive feel to what could have been a completely negative experience.

Teamworking

Adair (1986) tells us there are few things more satisfying in life than belonging to a really successful team. He defines a team as a group in which the individuals share a common aim and in which the jobs and skills of each member fit in with those of others. Successful organizations claim they owe their success to effective teamworking, because effective teams produce a far higher quality and quantity of work than individuals working on their own.

How a team is made-up is crucial to its success. One of the ways in which team working has been influenced is through the work of Belbin (1991), who assessed the effectiveness of management teams. By asking the question - 'what is the best mix of people to make an effective team?' - Belbin was able to identify eight team membership roles according to the personality of each team member. His work involved examining team inputs as well as outputs, and looking at the relationship between the two. The eight particular roles identified by Belbin have been summarized by Eggert (1994), who has added a ninth role. These are shown in Figure 5.12. alongside the 'allowable weaknesses' originally identified by Belbin.

The significance of all this means ideal teams can be created by mixing and balancing personality types. Belbin's work showed that when teams are made up of people with similar personality types, poor results occur. When there is competition for leadership, with too many co-ordinators and shapers who want to get things done, the team is less

BELBIN'S KEY TEAM - ROLES		
Type	**Typical Features and Positive Qualities (summarized by Eggert, 1994)**	**Allowable weaknesses (Belbin, 1991)**
Plant	Creative, imaginative, unorthodox, solves difficult problems	Up in clouds, inclined to disregard practical details
Resource Investigator	Extrovert, enthusiastic, communicative, explores opportunities, develops contacts	Liable to loose interest once initial fascination has passed
Co-ordinator	Mature, confident, good chairperson, clarifies, promotes decision-making, delegates well	No more than ordinary in intellectual or creative ability
Shaper	Challenging and dynamic, thrives on pressure, has drive and courage to overcome obstacles	Prone to provocation, irritation and impatience
Monitor - Evaluator	Sober, strategic and discerning, sees all options and judges accurately	Lacks inspiration or the ability to motivate others
Team Worker	Co-operative, mild, perceptive and diplomatic, listens, builds, averts friction, calms the waters	Indecisive at moments of crisis
Implementor	Disciplined, reliable, conservative and efficient, turns ideas into practical action.	Lack of flexibility, unresponsiveness to unproven ideas
Completer	Painstaking, conscientious, anxious, searching out errors and omissions, delivers on time	Tends to worry about small things. A reluctance to 'let go'
Specialist	Single minded, self standing, dedicated, provides knowledge and skill in rare supply	

Fig.5.12: 'Useful people to have in teams' showing their strengths and weakness

effective. If there is too much intellectual power this results in brilliant discussion but little performance, and the lack of intellectual power results in limitation of ideas and creativity. A weakness of Belbin's work is that it ignores gender differences in the way of working (Eggert, 1994). This may be of significance to midwifery managers because the majority of midwives are female, and the majority of senior doctors and senior managers are male. However, by building a balance in the team this will allow for individual weaknesses to be overcome by the natural strengths of others.

Team building

Adair (1986) believes that all leaders are team builders. Teams are always either improving or declining in effectiveness, therefore the work of the team builder is never done. He also asserts that few good leaders have quite the team they would wish for, just as few good teams have quite the leader they would like.

Selecting the right team is something that midwifery managers will have to believe in and must be committed to. It includes accepting the concept of 'balance' and the notion that 'nobody is perfect but a team can be'. Choosing the right team members includes assessing:

- their skills and contribution in decision-making, creativity and innovation
- their ability to listen to others
- their determination for high performance
- flexibility of mind

- integrity
- likeable personality
- eliminating non-starters - leaving out those not motivated, the non achievers and the disruptives.

Successful teams are dependent on the 'team mix' and also on the team leader to facilitate a balance of the team roles. The difficulty for midwifery managers is that they are not always in a position to choose the 'team mix', and have to develop the team they already have. Sometimes the assistance of an outside facilitator can help team members adapt a balance through mutually accepting their complementary roles. In this way members begin to accept different perspectives and interest within the team.

Factors for the successful development of teams

- Rewards should go to the team as a whole. According to Peters (1988) this is 'simple to state but tough to execute'. Team rewarding actually shifts the focus of evaluation to team performance, and includes pay and rewards.

- Members communicate with each other constantly. Effective decision-making springs from good communication.

- Members have a shared vision and purpose.

- Involving people outside the team, e.g. the users and the purchasers of maternity services, make them partners in the developing process. As Peters (1988) believes 'most innovation will come from these constituents, if you trust them they will trust you'. This concept was certainly the basis of *Changing Childbirth* (1993) which grew predominantly from the views and requirements of mothers in partnership with midwives.

Delegation

Good team work involves the delegation of work and tasks to others, who are able to do the work just as well, or better and quicker. Any member of the team can delegate work or tasks to others. As Hiley and Edis (1992) remind us 'delegation allows the delegating-person to get on with other work that may be a better use of their time and energy'. Delegation is about helping others to develop their abilities and making them answerable for results. It is about taking risks but not absolving responsibility. If a member of staff gets in a muddle it is the delegating-person who will still be liable. Delegation involves:

- assessing whether the person is capable of carrying out the work or requires training
- ensuring the person is able to identify problems and deal with them, and assess results
- having an appropriate monitoring system to reduce the risk of failure
- having patience with the person who may be slower and less efficient

- allowing the person time and space to get on with and complete the work without too much interference
- handing over favourite tasks and work as well as that least liked
- giving others more opportunities to take on more responsibility
- getting satisfaction from seeing others develop and grow.

Sometimes delegation does not succeed and can involve disappointments on both sides. A failure with one person does not mean delegation will fail with another. Although delegation involves some risk-taking the real benefits for midwifery managers and midwifery sisters are in releasing valuable time to undertake important activities, and at the same time developing motivated and responsible teams.

According to Peters (1988), although delegation has been a central topic in 'management text' for a long time now it is 'hot' and at the top of the list. He tells managers they must 'let go' and delegate or suffer the consequences of unacceptably slow action-taking. Effective delegation means really letting go to such an extent that it inspires others to take true and vigorous responsibility. Peters refers to this as 'the sine qua non of empowerment'. It involves:

- first a shared vision
- shared high standards
- reviewing every act of delegation to see you are really letting go
- monitoring casual remarks to those to whom you have delegated
- ensuring you don't inadvertently rescind the grant of autonomy.

Performance appraisal

Appraisal, consciously or unconsciously, is something everyone does. People appraise objects to assess their usefulness, value and quality. They appraise themselves and other people by judging behaviour, attitudes, personality and achievements. Organizational appraisal systems have been developed in an attempt to 'formalize these activities for the benefit of both the individual and the organization' (Torrington and Hall, 1991). Many terms have been used to mean appraisal and these include: performance assessment, performance evaluation, development review, job appraisal, individual assessment and individual performance review (IPR).

Most appraisals are carried out by the immediate superior. The advantage of this arrangement is that the immediate superior will be well acquainted with the person's job specification and goals, and will have the most information on how the person has performed. In practice, this is not always so. Francis and Woodcock (1982) observed that many organizations had badly designed appraisal systems but 'many well-defined systems did not meet their declared aims because of inappropriate actions by the participants'. Walton (1988) on the other hand recognized the far sightedness of the National Staff Committee (Nurses and Midwives) who championed appraisal systems within the NHS. He stressed the constructiveness of the joint discussion, but acknowledged a major barrier to the formalized system was the 'fear of paperwork'. In 1991 a survey conducted by the Institute of Health Services Management found 'the most striking feature of IPR was the diffidence with which some managers had embraced it' (Davies, 1991). The most worrying aspect of the report was that junior managers lacked clear objectives, had minimal feedback and had increased responsibility without clear control.

Purposes of performance appraisal

- to provide a mechanism for formal assessment of an individual's performance, by assessing the accomplishment of goals and standards in the job
- to provide an individual with feedback on performance, standards of practice and variances in performances - strengths and weaknesses.
- to assess and review an individual's continuing education, training and development needs
- to plan and agree future goals and standards to be accomplished
- to consider future career development and opportunities.

The appraisal process

Midwifery managers and midwifery sisters have the responsibility to initiate appraisal discussions with their staff. Appraisals should not be left until the last minute or carried out in a hurried manner.

SETTING GOALS AND STANDARDS

Before a performance appraisal can begin the member of staff and midwifery manager must have previously reached a mutual agreement of the goals and standards to be accomplished in the job. If expectations are not clear and mutually understood, performance will be difficult to accomplish.

PLANNING THE APPRAISAL

Prior to conducting the appraisal the midwifery manager will:

- review the job requirements
- review the goals and standards previously discussed and agreed with the individual
- review the individual's skills, training and experience, previous job performance and any special qualifications
- evaluate the individual's job performance and standards for the period being appraised
- note any differences in performance and provide specific examples for discussion
- consider any appropriate education, training, and development required.

PRIOR TO THE APPRAISAL THE MEMBER OF STAFF WILL:

- carry out a 'self appraisal' of their performance in the job, standards achieved, strengths and weaknesses, areas for development and education and training needs
- make a record of their assessment for discussion at the appraisal. This can be written in the individual's own words, or by completing a form specially designed

for the purpose. In either event the individual's 'self assessment' will remain their own property. Its main purpose is to help the individual focus on their performance and provide concrete information for discussion during the appraisal.

CONDUCTING THE APPRAISAL:
- the discussion should be held in private, away from noise and interruptions
- the midwifery manager summarizes the purpose of appraisal, agrees the structure for the meeting, checks the 'self assessment' has been done and establishes a mutual understanding.
- the member of staff is asked to review their work and accomplishments over the past year. This allows the appraisee to select where to begin and gain confidence.
- the midwifery manager offers her views, shows where there are agreements and disagreements and explains why
- differences between expectations and results of the appraisee and appraiser are explored and disagreement resolved
- future goals are assessed and agreed
- the midwifery manager summarizes in a positive manner, giving the appraisee opportunity to react, question and add any further suggestions.

FOLLOWING THE APPRAISAL MEETING:
- the appraisal form is completed and signed by both the member of staff and midwifery manager.

THE SUCCESS OF APPRAISAL DEPENDS ON:
- managers understanding what appraisal can achieve and visibly 'owning' the system
- staff understanding what appraisal is about and not confusing it with disciplinary action.
- openness and participation during the appraisal discussions
- training managers in the appraisal process and how to appraise and conduct interviews.
- monitoring agreed 'action plans' and ensuring they take place
- appraisal systems reflecting both the needs of the organization and individuals.

Absenteeism

Absenteeism is a problem. Left uncontrolled it will not improve. In fact absenteeism unchecked will get worse and cause extreme harm to the efficiency and success of an organization. Tylczak (1991) maintains that a 'business that has fifteen per cent of its employees out at any time will almost certainly compromise its profits, productivity and performance'.

Most people will, at some time or other, find themselves unable to work for reasons that are genuine. Usually this is due to sickness or accident, and occasionally due to serious illness or death of a close family member. Rarely travel problems due to adverse weather conditions or public transport difficulties may prevent a person getting in to the workplace. Indirect forms of absenteeism are staff who persistently arrive late for work and leave early.

Short term absenteeism that is taken frequently, in odd days and without an appropriate reason is a serious problem. Usually this indicates that a person has planned an absence intentionally. Argyle (1979) describes this as voluntary absenteeism and says it occurs 'simply because workers would rather do something else than come to work'. Some of the causes of short term absenteeism are;

- lack of job satisfaction
- work related stress
- personal emotional difficulties
- childcare difficulties
- alcohol and drug abuse.

A study commissioned by the Health Education Authority in 1995 *Health At Work in the NHS* showed that the percentage of time taken off sick by staff ranged from one per cent to eleven per cent, with an average percentage of five, the national average being three and a half. There were wide differences in the amount of sick time taken by various groups of health workers and one NHS Trust reported a sickness and absenteeism rate of six per cent for nurses and midwives but one per cent for medical staff. However, the authors did accept the findings may have been faulty because of the wide discrepancies in the way statistics are recorded and used across the NHS.

Taylor (1995) estimates that the cost to the average District General Hospital of staff going off sick is £1.4 million. Further she states that female nurses and midwives take more time than women employed in other sectors in the country.

Effects of sickness and absenteeism

Absenteeism causes problems because the work still has to be done and it affects other staff as they have to take on extra responsibilities leading to an increased workload. This leads to negative attitudes being formed against the 'absent colleague' such as exasperation, resentment and loss of respect.

How to manage absenteeism

- have a monitoring system for reporting and recording all staff absences
- encourage staff to discuss their health problems in confidence with the midwifery manager and to use the Occupational Health Department more readily
- when there is a problem of absenteeism accept it exists
- recognize absenteeism is also a morale problem
- analyse the causes, the reasons individuals give as to why they are absent from work, and the pattern of absenteeism across the maternity services
- consider alternative solutions to resolve the problem

- share the plan of action with staff, give positive reinforcement, measure results and get feedback from staff
- support and help staff who are on genuine sick leave.

A CASE EXAMPLE FOR MANAGING SICKNESS AND ABSENTEEISM

The problem: A maternity services unit with two postnatal wards had an absenteeism problem. Ward one had an average sickness-absenteeism rate of five days per person per year, and ward two had an average of nine days per person per year. Both wards were managed by the same midwifery manager, who had been monitoring the worsening situation in the second ward.

The solution: The midwifery manager decided to design a 'feedback letter' to send to the staff. Those in the lower ten per cent of sick leave were sent a letter acknowledging the manager's appreciation of their excellent attendance record and thanking them. Staff in the upper ten per cent were sent a letter telling them they had been off sick more than the average member of staff. Whilst it emphasized they were not expected to report for work when ill, they were urged to exercise good judgement. The letter ended by hoping the forthcoming year would find them in better health.

The result: The 'Hawthorne effect' took over and the sickness rate improved in the upper ten per cent. The 'Hawthorne effect' according to Tylczak (1991) is 'when managers pay attention to staff, they will improve'. Handy (1993) contends the 'Hawthorne effect' may result from staff experiencing a new way of working, of 'being the focus of managerial and research attention' which generates much of the improvement in morale and output.

Preventing absenteeism

High staff morale is a key to lowering absentee rates. Midwifery managers and midwifery sisters can ensure morale is raised and maintained by:

OBSERVING THEIR OWN ATTENDANCE BEHAVIOUR

- are they always punctual
- do others always know where they are
- are they contactable in an emergency
- are absenteeism practices applied equitably and fairly.

GIVING POSITIVE FEEDBACK

- is positive reinforcement offered
- are staff rewarded for good attendance records
- are absentee issues dealt with positively
- are individual and group successes acknowledged
- is appreciation sincere and honest.

Recently, some NHS Trusts have reported providing financial incentives for staff, by linking bonus pay offers to improved sickness levels (Taylor, 1995). Incentive payments applied to each clinical directorate will give staff opportunity to share in savings made from the reduction of costs due to sickness. Opponents to incentive payments believe these will increase staff stress levels and ill-health and that an improvement in absenteeism is firmly linked to the way staff are appreciated and managed. A combination of positive absenteeism management and incentive bonuses would seem to be the way forward.

Time management

Life revolves around time, and time governs our lives. The concept of time is a constant phenomenon because as Mackenzie states each one of us 'has all the time there is' (La Monica, 1994), but few of us ever has enough time.

Midwifery managers and midwives should pay particular attention to time because time costs money for the Maternity Services and the NHS Trust. As Mackenzie accurately observed (La Monica, 1994) 'time is a resource that cannot be stockpiled or accumulated, and it cannot be turned on or off'. Drucker (La Monica, 1994) said time is so important that unless it is managed, nothing else can be managed. As the hours at work are unlikely to increase for midwifery managers this means that available time has to be used as effectively as possible. Activities have been categorized into time wasters and time consumers, and Lakein (La Monica, 1994) estimated that eighty per cent of time is wasted, leaving only twenty per cent of time for important issues.

Methods of time management

Time management is not an end in itself, but a means to an end in order to get a little more time out of the time given. There is no magic formula, but when time management is successful the ratio of effort to payoff is high, which contributes to cost effectiveness.

Midwifery managers can improve their management of time by:

- developing 'time management' techniques - for dealing with time-wasters, self examination and analysis of time and methods for further improvement
- setting and meeting goals - so that time management provides a way for high achievement for self and others
- planning and prioritizing activities - so that the important issues are dealt with as a priority. This has to be redefined on a daily basis to accommodate any changing pattern of needs.

How to develop techniques for the better management of time

- Examine yourself and commit yourself to improving. If unwilling to commit yourself ask yourself why, and concentrate on converting yourself from a reluctant to enthusiastic manager of time
- Learn to say no - Other people always have a priority that another must do. These people surround us. You must be able to sort out the important i.e. assignments with a high pay off, from the unimportant with a low pay-off. Agree to do the former, and say 'no' to the latter without feeling and showing guilt.

- Plan the use of time. List your responsibilities, choose priorities and plan how you will achieve them. Develop a daily, weekly and monthly 'to do list' and check off progress. This is a self-reinforcement technique for further accomplishment and motivation. Do not include unimportant small details on your list, but allow for flexibility, especially on you weekly and monthly lists.
- Record how time is used. Use a time-analysis worksheet, to see how your time has been used. This will raise an awareness of your own behaviour, by making the abstract concrete (La Monica, 1994).
- Use prime time to its advantage. Most of us have a time in the day which we know is our prime time. During this time we are at our best, and work is usually easier to accomplish. Block this time off and use it - this will probably be the time when eighty per cent of your work will get done effectively. Look after your prime time and protect it.
- Programme 'small blocks of time'. We all need time and space to think. Plan small blocks of time in your day for this, and let people know you do not wish to be disturbed. Intrusions are big time wasters and cost you thinking time.
- Avoid filling your day with only the things you like doing. It is easy to fill one's day with jobs one likes at the expense of jobs that are less enjoyable, but nevertheless as important. Avoidance of work we do not like doing, and filling our with other things, is very common. Examine your approach to work, and question whether your own skills and the skills of others are being used to their greatest advantage at all times.
- Manage meetings effectively. According to the Industrial Society (1982) most meetings are a waste of time. People often wonder why they are there and find meetings a demoralising experience. Get the most out of meetings for yourself and others. The most productive and efficient meetings are those that are well planned and are timely (see Meetings - Chapter 7).

Summary

Recent NHS reforms have had a major impact on the way resources are managed. Contractual funding has separated the purchasers of health care from the providers and resource management has given clinicians more responsibility for the way resources are used. Demands for an increase in resources for health care will always be infinite, but NHS funding is finite. Hence the government's drive for 'value for money'.

Understanding the nature of primary and secondary resources is essential for midwifery managers, especially as these are associated with productivity, economy, efficiency and effectiveness.

A retrospective look at the Resource Management Iniative (1987) provides comprehension of the events that led to the present Clinical Directorate structure. Although various Directorate structures have been tried, the duumvirate arrangement is currently fashionable. Resource management involves clinicians in management and utilizes fully integrated information systems to support clinical and management decision-making. The benefits are greater efficiency and more responsive management at the level of clinical care.

Effective human resource management is crucial for the provision of high standards in the NHS. Despite the slogan 'people are our most important asset', staff frequently remain undervalued and undertrained in many organizations. The drive for 'value for money' has forced NHS Trusts to choose whether to adopt a 'hard or soft' approach to human resource management.

Current human resource management focuses on demand rather than supply, and on developing strategies to meet the requirements of the NHS Trust. Employee cooperation is essential, and this can be achieved by creating the right culture, and through remuneration packages, teamworking and management development. Patterns emerging in NHS Trust Human Resource Strategies show a more independent approach to employment practices, the use of short term contracts and an emphasis on training and development.

Recruitment and selection of the right staff for the Maternity Services is one of the biggest challenges facing midwifery managers in the late 1990s. Using effective recruitment processes managers will be enabled to appoint staff with the right knowledge, skills and motivation to do the job.

Successful organizations claim they owe their success to effective team working. Effective teams produce a far higher quality and quantity of work than individuals working on their own. Belbin's study on the composition of effective management teams provides an insight into what constitutes a balanced team. Selecting the appropriate team members, team building and the successful management of teams are all dependent on the team leader. Team working involves delegation. Delegation is about helping others to develop their abilities and to be answerable for their results. Delegation involves taking risks, knowing how to 'let go' but not absolving responsibility.

Performance appraisals assess how staff perform in their jobs. They involve individual's setting and agreeing their own goals with their manager and formally assessing their performance. Successful appraisals are dependent on staff and managers understanding the system, openness during the appraisal discussion and ensuring agreed action takes place.

Absenteeism is a problem. Left uncontrolled it will not improve. Most absences are genuine and are due to sickness or accident but short term absences taken frequently and without good reason require investigation. Absenteeism affects other staff because the work still has to be done. Managing absenteeism and maintaining high staff mo ale are the keys to lowering absentee rates.

Time is a resource, and time costs money. If time is not managed properly, nothing else can be managed. Time management involves developing techniques for organizing time better, setting and meeting goals and planning and prioritizing activities.

CHAPTER SIX

Stressors in the Work Environment

'It is easy to assume that the National Health Service, which exists to treat and prevent illness, is a healthy place to work - but this is not so.'
(Harriet Harman, 1988)

Creating a culture that is open and responsive, and a work environment that is healthy and safe is the aim of every National Health Service employer. Health and safety is bound in law, and employers hold a responsibility for safeguarding the health, safety and welfare of staff as is reasonably practical. This includes providing a safe working environment, having safe practices in place e.g. correct lifting procedures, infection control, and making sure staff take on a responsibility for themselves through education and training.

Despite these safeguards, stressors still develop in the workplace. Often these are associated with or result from the specialized work staff do, and the people they come in contact with. This chapter includes four work stressors that concern midwives and looks at positive ways of dealing with them. These will be of particular interest to midwifery managers and midwifery sisters for the formulation policies, and for education and training.

Baby snatching

'If someone is determined to take a baby, the chances are they may very well get one'. (Royal College of Midwives, 1995)

The kidnapping of three babies from Maternity Units during the past five years has amazed and terrified the general public. In each case the baby snatcher has been able to enter a Maternity Unit, gain the confidence of one of the parents and take away their baby. The first baby snatcher posed as a health visitor, the second dressed as a nurse and asked the father to hand over his newborn baby for a 'hearing test' and the third befriended the mother, and whilst leaving the mother in another room, smuggled her baby out of the postnatal ward in a shopping bag. In each case the baby snatcher has been a woman, who has not been motivated to kidnap by maternal desire but, as Lee-Potter (1995) aptly puts it, by a 'selfish drive to hang on to the man in her life, and to use the baby as a bribe to keep him'.

Midwives and other health workers are destroyed by baby snatches. According to John Raburn Jr, Vice President of the USA Centre for Missing and Exploited Children (1994) 'nurses are often more traumatised than the victims of hospital baby abduction'. He says staff are inevitably traumatised, and when a baby snatch occurs they are the real victims, as the parents appear to make a quicker recovery once reunited with their baby. Following a baby snatch, midwives and the staff closely involved will suffer a variety of after-effects, and the midwifery manager will need to be supportive as well as objective in obtaining details surrounding the incident. Early reporting of the incident to senior managers is essential and working closely with the police will be necessary. Staff will need to be helped to cooperate but must not made to feel guilty. Those staff who experience long term after-effects will require professional counselling.

Action to deter baby snatchers

Although midwifery managers need to ensure safety and protection for all those who use and work in the Maternity Unit, they must guard against the 'Fortress Mentality' as described by Hunt (1994). The fear of baby snatching can so often be out of proportion to its actual occurrence, but preventing it must still be taken seriously. The challenge for midwifery managers is to calm people's fears by responding positively and involving them in a number of practices which can act as a deterrent, and make the Maternity Unit as secure as possible. As Prescott (1995) reminds us, if security warnings are too stark they can leave parents fearful, when the actual risks are extremely low. High security can be achieved without an oppressive atmosphere and there are a number of choices, which may include all or some of the following:

- security procedures and practices - continually reviewing and updating procedures to reflect any changes necessary to ensure the safety of mothers, babies and staff.
- staff to wear identity badges, including other health professionals who visit mothers and babies in the Maternity Unit.
- electronic tagging of babies, which set off an alarm if the baby is taken outside authorized areas. Unfortunately reports suggest these sometimes fail if wet, and also they can be snipped off with scissors.
- coded entry systems to wards and departments for regular midwifery and obstetric medical staff. All other health workers and visitors being required to gain entry by ringing a bell or via an integrated telephone or video system.
- 24 hour hospital security guards who patrol the site and are available to staff through alarm systems and contact points.
- surveillance cameras or videos in the hospital and grounds.
- 'Hospital Watch Scheme' - a voluntary arrangement where designated staff in various areas of the Maternity Unit and the hospital keep a look-out for unusual occurrences and report these immediately to the security guard or hospital porter and the manager on duty.
- staff vigilance - especially as the profile of a baby snatcher is almost the same in every case and they frequently visit the maternity unit just prior to the abduction. Cameras and baby tagging are very effective when combined with staff vigilance.
- leaflets for mothers - which provide basic advice on safety and security for themselves and their baby. These can be of simple design, clear and practical,

aimed at helping new mothers to follow sensible precautions without causing unnecessary alarm. The aim is awareness, not to cause anxiety.
- staff training - mainly in small groups, encouraging midwives to discuss the whole issue of baby snatching and its prevention.

The decision as to which security measures to use must be firmly based on need. It is not acceptable to overreact and introduce an assortment of 'hard security systems' if they are not required. Most importantly the midwifery manager needs to remember that the best security measures are those that blend with the culture and ethos of the of Maternity Unit and the NHS Trust, but at the same time protect the occupants of the hospital and the staff who provide their care.

Complaints

'Effective complaints procedures are the mark of a healthy corporate organization.' (Editorial. *Nursing Times,* May,1994.)

No one likes complaints, and this is especially so when the complaint is made directly against a midwife concerning her clinical practice, criticizing her for something she did, or did not do, in the course of caring for others.

Since the introduction of *The Patients Charter* (1991), there is no doubt that expectations of people using the Health Service have risen, and this is reflected in the increase in the number of complaints. Dealing with complaints is an extremely sensitive issue in a highly emotive area such as childbirth, where the expectations of mothers and their families are for the birth of a live healthy baby, and where women want more control surrounding their baby's birth. Sometimes the complainant is a bereaved parent, which has driven them to complain and further adds to their distress. Complaints must be investigated speedily. Every complaint must be dealt with sensitively and effectively, so that lessons can be learnt to avoid similar situations. For many midwives though the stress placed upon them during an investigation is devastating. Even if, following the investigation, they are exonerated they often experience long term after-effects, resulting in a lack of confidence in their professional practice. Additionally, some midwives are worried about the increase in litigation claims associated with childbirth, which can stretch on for years before the case is heard.

Main reasons given for complaints against professional staff
- inadequate treatment
- standard of care below that expected
- unsatisfactory attitude of staff
- poor, insensitive and inadequate communications
- failure to diagnose, or late diagnosis
- errors in procedures
- inadequate resource availability
- prolonged length of wait for treatment
- absence of helpful information or guidance

Possible effects of complaints

MOTHERS

- consider making a complaint can be off-putting
- can feel distressed during a complaint investigation and in need of help
- are often afraid that making a complaint will influence her care in the future
- frequently end up resenting the Maternity Service and all those concerned with her care
- fear being involved in a legal 'battle'.

MIDWIVES

- are disappointed and concerned that their professional competence has been questioned and criticized
- suffer anxiety; fear, anger and depression
- develop a defensive attitude to those trying to investigate the complaint
- become reluctant to provide written reports or 'statements' concerning the events surrounding the complaint
- have difficulty in articulating problems and incidents leading to the complaint.

MIDWIFERY MANAGERS

- have a need to investigate and resolve complaints quickly
- are dependent on the open responsiveness of midwives
- have pressure from senior managers/Chief Executive to keep within timescale and to resolve the complaint satisfactorily
- disappointment
- are frequently involved in lengthy drawn-out complaint processes which are difficult to resolve and are distressing to all concerned.

There is no doubt the mechanism for handling complaints in the National Health Service is inappropriate. It is cumbersome and bureaucratic, a top to bottom approach, and one in which midwives feel threatened and midwifery managers feel frustrated. The present complaints system is embodied in the Patients Charter being one of the 'New Rights' added April 1992 and reads as follows:

> 'to have any complaint about NHS services - whoever provides them - investigated, and to receive a full and prompt written reply from the chief executive of your health authority or your hospital. If you are still unhappy, you will be able to take the case up with the Health Service Commissioner'.

In April 1993, the National Association of Health Authorities and Trusts (NAHAT) in their Report 'Complaints Do Matter' called for a more user friendly and speedier complaints procedure. The report recognized the considerable dissatisfaction in the National Health Service among health professionals and the organizations representing users of the service. It called for a substantial change in the way that National Health Service complaints are dealt with.

Managing complaints effectively

- Every complaint, verbal and written, must be taken seriously.

- Complaints are best dealt with at the level where they arise and must be timely.

- The 'Named Midwife' and 'Associate Midwife' arrangement will empower mothers and midwives to relate more openly with each other. If there are difficulties or dissatisfactions these can be more easily dealt with at, or near to the time, of occurrence.

- Midwives will need to develop skills of awareness and sensitivity to pick up feelings of dissatisfaction and discontent, and to be able to raise these with the mother and her partner, so they can be resolved.

- Verbal complaints either direct or 'indirect' still need to be investigated and the mother kept informed of progress until a response is available.

- Printed information in the 'Mothers Own Notes' can tell her that if a problem or complaint cannot be resolved with her 'named' or 'associate midwife', then this can be referred to the midwifery manager, and how she can go about doing this.

- During more formal investigations of a complaint the midwifery manager and the midwives concerned should make personal contact with the complainant, to discuss and attempt to resolve the complaint.

- Complainants are entitled to:
  - be told how their complaint will be handled
  - be advised in writing of the conclusion reached and the reasons for this
  - an apology when a complaint is upheld and brief details of any action being taken to improve the service for the future.

- Continuing Education and In-service Training should be provided for midwives in:
  - communication and listening skills and questioning techniques
  - skills in awareness and how to assess a situation
  - how to handle and investigate complaints
  - how to write reports and 'statements' and accept them as an integral part of the complaint procedure.
  - working in an open organizational culture.

- Leaflets for mothers should be simple and user-friendly and include the following:
  - how to make your views known
  - how to go about making a verbal or written complaint
  - how a complaint is handled.

- Monitoring and publicising statistics about the way complaints have been handled in the Maternity Services and their outcomes. Acknowledging any changes in procedure or practice as a result of the investigation. To keep complaints in perspective a useful way is to concurrently monitor and publicize 'Letters of Compliment' so that a balance between the two can be seen.

The future

New measures, due to be implemented 1 April 1996, will give lay people a major part in adjudicating clinical complaints about midwives, nurses and other health professionals. The new NHS Complaints Procedure will consist of two stages - stage one will be the internal investigation and stage two will only be introduced if the internal investigation does not satisfy the complainant. Clinical and administrative complaints will need to be resolved and settled quickly by NHS Trusts, but if a solution is not reached and the complainant is still dissatisfied, then Non Executives of the Trust can convene an independent panel. This will be chaired by a lay person and be expected to reach a decision with access to appropriate clinical advice. As a final resort, the remit of the Health Service Commissioner will be expanded to cover clinical as well as administrative procedures.

The aim of the new NHS Complaints Procedure is for a 'single, simple and speedy' system for people complaining about the health service. It promises to be a fairer arrangement for mothers and midwives, but the onus will certainly be on midwives to act swiftly and attempt to resolve complaints in the first instance. The challenge for the midwifery manager will, of course, be to agree and implement effective practices and procedures, but more significantly to facilitate and guide midwives to deal with complaints as soon as they arise.

Stress at work

> 'My candle burns at both ends, Oh! what a lovely sight. But oh! my foe and oh! my friends, It will not last the night.' (Anon)

Stress became a fashionable word in the 1980s. Tension, and to some extent stress, can be positive forces, and according to Nelson (1992) no organization could operate effectively, or at all, without them. Some people thrive on stress, enjoying the stimulus to perform at their peak, whilst others find it to be harmful and destructive. Stress as a negative force, is usually used to describe 'unpleasant feelings of too much pressure and a subsequent inability to cope'. Negativity is destructive.

A useful working definition of stress, has been produced by Bond (1988), who describes stress as 'an experience of unpleasant over-or-under-stimulation, as defined by the individual in question, that actually or potentially leads to ill health'.

Stress is a major occupational hazard. Rogers and Salvage (1988) estimate it is responsible for more time off work than accidents. They assert that many of the harmful stressors in our working lives are the direct result of the failure of employers to regard the health and welfare of their staff as a top priority. Also they tell us of the irony that has been noted about the National Health Service, that despite its commitment to improving people's health, it is no better an employer in this respect than many others. Midwifery managers must have a working knowledge about stress and how it can manifest, but they also need to be able to recognize that the potential for stress exists between the interface of personal and home life, work and the style of management used. We are reminded by Nelson (1992) that workers are 'twenty-four hour' people in that their domestic values and pressures affect them at work and vice versa. Often pressures from one area will exacerbate problems in another. This is particularly true when workloads are high and deadlines are approaching at work or when there are problems or illness at home.

Reactions to stress

A person's reaction to stress is a primitive one, used by our early ancestors and known as the fright:fight:flight response. When in immediate danger, the instant response is a natural body-reaction which is necessary to enable a person to fight and overcome the danger, or to run away and escape for self-preservation. When constant tension and continued stress is present there is no outlet. Bodily changes remain prepared and ready for fight or to run, yet the body is unable to do so. Consequently, a number of physiological and psychological warning signals occur when stress has reached an uncontrollable level. These can cause problems when the conditions have to be suffered continuously. In western medicine only now do doctors refer to stress as a cause of illness, but as Mole (1993) reflects 'it is a strange paradox that although GPs often cite stress as the cause of a person's complaint, the main medical textbooks do not even list it in their sections on the cause of disease'. Each person has their own pattern of responding signals which are not the same in everyone, but will usually include one or more of the following symptoms:

Physiological
- headache - throbbing head or pain spreading over back of head
- grinding teeth, twitching eyes, tremulous voice
- hyperventilation, palpitations, breathlessness, chest discomfort
- nail-biting, damaged cuticles, twiddling thumbs
- indigestion, vomiting, diarrhoea, diabetes, backache
- frequency of micturition - skin rashes, tiredness
- sweating, trembling, fainting, insomnia

Psychological
- increase in smoking, increase in alcohol consumption
- increase or decrease in appetite
- inability or continual desire and capacity to sleep
- depression, absent-mindedness, lack of concentration
- loss of sex drive, irritability, impulsiveness

Other feelings related to stress
- worthlessness, anxiety, anger, guilt

Professional burnout

Stress is one of the principal causes of human breakdown at work, which is referred to as 'professional burnout'. The term 'burnout' was first contrived by the psychoanalyst Dr Herbert Freudenberger (Bond, Holland and Lamplugh, 1988) who described it as a syndrome of 'physical and emotional exhaustion, involving the development of negative self-concepts, negative attitudes towards work or job, and a loss of interest and concern for the feelings of others'. Although 'burnout' only occurs in a relatively small number of people, it is worth describing because the effect of one person experiencing the condition can lower the morale in the workplace.

Bond and Holland (1988) describe four stages leading to burnout which include:

1. Feelings of doubt and uncertainty about coping with a job, especially when newly appointed to a post. There is a tendency to be overconscientious and to overwork, displaying lots of energy and enthusiasm.

2. Feelings of irritation, tiredness, anxiety and frustration develop. There is a tendency to experience a sense of stagnation, like 'beating ones head against the wall' or 'never getting to the top of the hill'. Everything is dreadful and unrelenting, and there is an inclination to blame others for what is happening.

3. Increasing periods of anger, disappointment and resentment occur. Feelings of failure and dissatisfaction with work predominate. Additionally there will be increasing feelings of guilt, lowering of self-esteem, thoughts of inadequacy and a sense of apathy, such as 'why bother?'

4. Profound personal distress. Physiological and psychological symptoms materialize, and there is a tendency of 'not wanting to go to work'. Feelings of complete failure and non-achievement are experienced.

Shine (1991) gives an interesting account of 'burnout', which she attributes to the energy and physical body not working together. She lists a number of enlightening characteristics plus advancing signs of 'burnout', some of which will be familiar to, and cannot be ignored by those working in management positions. These are:

*   ambitious: always working hard
*   not afraid of overtime, taking responsibility or promotion
*   suddenly with a dawning that 'exactive' standards have to be maintained for the rest of ones working life. This leads to a feeling of being 'trapped'
*   younger ambitious workers are all around and full of energy
*   feelings of tiredness begin - work isn't going as well as it used to
*   negativity has crept in with worries about work but must pretend that everything is fine.

Ultimately 'burnout' leads to:

*   job dissatisfaction, reduced commitment to work
*   withdrawal, sickness and absence
*   lowering of morale in the workplace.

Those suffering from 'burnout' will need:

- long term support
- referral to the NHS Trust Occupational Health Department
- professional counselling.

Causes of stress at work

Many reasons causing stress in the workplace are not, of course, specific to the job. Because personal life and work are intrinsically linked they impinge on each other and vice versa. Other factors prevalent in society can also create stress, especially among a predominantly female workforce as in midwifery. These are:

- Organizing childcare: This is still considered the responsibility of women who have to take time off work when their child is ill.

- Caring for dependants: Looking after a sick, elderly or disabled relative is usually carried out in addition to paid employment.

- 'Running' the home: Household chores; shopping and organizing meals are usually left to women.

- General increase in the pace of life: Cramming far too much into each day with little time for relaxation and spiritual reflections

Some of the work induced stress situations are preventable, and the midwifery manager should be able to reduce these pressures through sound organizational management. Nevertheless, there will always be some staff who will still feel stressed whatever improvements are made, but at least by working with them pressures should be reduced to a manageable level. The main reasons given by staff which attribute to stress are:

Workload
- usually referred to as the major cause of occupational stress
- pressure to increase quantitative workload within contracts
- a perception of little or no real control of workload
- estimating there are not enough staff to do the work.

Lack of physical resources
- scarcity of the correct equipment to do the job well
- working environment and building design not always conducive for providing high standards of care.

Working arrangements
- odd timing and variation of shifts to provide a 24 hour service
- on-call duties - especially call-out during night hours

- working long stretches without a break
- working an early shift following after a late shift.

Professional pressures

- when especially when dealing with difficult and distressing situations in midwifery practice, such as serious complications, neonatal abnormalities and bereavement
- midwives suppressing their feelings and hiding their emotions
- inadequate role preparation for work changes and insecurity about expectations and performance in the new role.
- increased pressure to develop and advance professionally through continuing education and to progress one's career
- an increase in professional complaints and possible litigation.

Change

- in itself is stressful
- uncertainty about NHS changes and doubts about whether the new management arrangement is providing a caring health service
- the future position and status of midwives and nurses within the new health service, especially in relation to doctors and managers.
- implementing *Changing Childbirth* (1993) recommendations and how these can be completed within the present resources and given timescale.

Management pressures (not exclusive)

- when outcome of negotiations and agreements are extremely important
- confronting or dismissing a member of staff
- dealing with severe critical feedback
- not achieving or finishing assignments or seeing the results of personal and committed 'hard' work
- finishing things so fast there is no time to reflect on what has been done.

Ways of reducing stress in the workplace

Matching staffing and skill levels to the workload

This can be done by planning the workload in a ward, department or community area as objectively as possible. This is not an easy assignment, especially as demands to increase output come from many different sources. These range from the mothers (for themselves and their babies), medical staff, midwifery managers, senior trust managers, finance officers, purchasers and the midwives themselves. It is a fact that many midwives say they feel guilty and experience stress at the end of a shift, especially when they feel they have not been able to provide a high standard of service for mothers and babies in their care.

By planning priorities midwifery managers and midwifery sisters take on a share of the responsibility for what has been accomplished, but more significantly for what has not been achieved. In this way the standards and quality of work can be controlled by evaluation and planning. Through agreeing, setting and owning standards midwives and their managers will begin to achieve a balance between quality and quantity. Not only will this form a basis for measuring workload and the quality of care, it will enable midwifery managers to be more objective with decision-making, skill-mix reviews and will facilitate them in their bids for additional resources. Most importantly, it will help staff to establish priorities in their work, in the knowledge that not all work required can be accomplished at once.

Smoothing out peaks of workload

Peaks of activity are not unusual or uncommon in providing a maternity service, despite good planning. Acute stress can be caused by a sudden peak in workload, and the midwifery manager can smooth the peaks and reduce stress by allocating additional staff or resources. Maintaining a 'Midwives Bank' gives midwives who do not want to work full-time or on a permanent basis, the opportunity to work when needed, on a casual basis. The effectiveness of a 'Midwives Bank' is to ensure midwives will be available at short notice during certain periods and that they are up-to-date and competent in their professional practice. In situations of short-term staff shortages due to sickness but with a low workload, a standby arrangement' of midwives who are prepared to work additional hours if required is usually adequate. It is especially effective for such departments as labour suite and neonatal unit. Those on standby must be midwives and staff who currently work in these specialized areas to ensure a high standard of practical skills.

Another way of dealing with a sudden peak in workload is for the midwifery manager or midwifery sister to make a conscious decision with the staff involved of what work should be completed and what can be left undone. Generally it is acceptable to defer some work to another time, but if this is left to backlog this in itself can be a cause of stress.

Open communications

By using sound and timely communication processes the midwifery manager can keep staff fully informed, involved and motivated. Moreover staff need to feel valued. Acknowledging individual staff members for their new ideas and innovations in practice is good, but the contribution staff make on a day-to-day basis must be recognized. This can be acknowledged during staff meetings, and on an individual basis during appraisal and staff development reviews.

Personal rationalization

Encouraging staff to be more self-aware about stress, its causes and to use preventive techniques, will help them cope more effectively with stress. These can range from relaxation, practical exercises and meditation; learning and developing confidence, assertiveness and sharing their problems and feelings with others in a secure confident atmosphere. The midwife may choose to use one of these techniques, or may have various approaches.

Peer group support

Midwives can help reduce their work-related stress levels through participating in open discussions and expressing their feelings with other midwives. This can be achieved through small groups of midwives meeting, usually in work time, to share experiences associated with work, how they felt at the time and may still be feeling. Through open discussion others will join in, so everyone has a chance to contribute and share their own experiences. The knowledge that midwives are not alone in their feelings will be reassuring. It has to be emphasized, however, that 'support groups' need to be structured otherwise they could turn into a 'grousing' session which could cause more stress.

Formal meetings

These can be held regularly by midwifery managers, midwifery sisters and or midwifery educationalists, specifically to discuss work related issues and incidents, so that feelings can be aired. They should take the form of a discussion and be constructive. Therefore the leader or facilitator needs to be experienced in the relevant skills. These skills can be developed through reading and in-service education. Occasionally, a skilled external facilitator can be invited to lead a discussion, which may encourage some staff to express their feelings more freely. However, a good rapport between an 'outside' leader and the midwifery manager must be first established, for planning the session and effective outcomes.

Education and training

Current pre registration education at diploma and degree level, through an integrative approach, provides knowledge and practice for the art and science of midwifery. It also prepares midwives to become critical, analytical and creative practitioners. Student midwives learn about the changing social and health needs, behaviourism and about stress. This preparation should at least provide midwives with the necessary requirements to recognize stress in themselves and others, and how to deal with it.

Midwives educated at traditional certificate level did not have the opportunity to learn about stress in the curriculum. Additionally, they were prepared for midwifery practice in a culture that did not encourage an overt expression of feelings. Today they can learn about the management of stress through continuing and in-service education in the form of study days, workshops and courses leading to a Higher Award in Professional Midwifery Studies.

Culture of the organization

Creating a culture to one that is open, supportive and honest will help focus on the beliefs and values of the staff, the 'norms' of behaviour and will reflect the style of management. A culture where managers and staff work consistently together will have a shared and inspired vision for the future. Through transformational leadership managers will empower others to be their own leaders.

Creating the right culture for the Maternity Service is a continuous process. Through day-to-day communication, formal and informal meetings, in-service and continuing education, staff can be facilitated towards changing their organizational culture to one that is 'sharing and caring'. As each member of staff contributes to the organizational culture midwifery managers and midwifery sisters have a particular responsibility to reshape attitudes and beliefs. (Also see Chapter 2 'Transforming Leadership' and Chapter 4 'Understanding Corporate Culture').

The challenge of change

There must be acceptance that everything changes and that change involves a degree of uncertainty. Roger and Nash (1995) point out that every change requires a transition, and stress arises if the transition is resisted or not made at all. They link stress to personality. The way a person copes with stress is dependent on their 'locus of control' and tolerance to ambiguity. Research with locus of control suggests that having an 'internal' orientation helps to protect or buffer people against the impact of stress, whereas those having an 'external' orientation tend to feel helpless and at the mercy of factors not under their control. Tolerance to ambiguity is a measure of how 'accepting a person is' to uncertainty. Those with a high tolerance will be able to accept a state of uncertainty and therefore make the transition to a new state. Training workshops on 'The Challenge of Change' will help staff understand their own personalities, why they react as they do, and how to look at change more as a challenge which brings about opportunity. Thus stress associated with change will be reduced.

Networking

This has been very successfully used in the USA. It is an effective way for midwifery managers and midwifery sisters to keep in touch, and link up with other midwives across the country in similar positions of work. Through informal networks midwives can communicate with each other, offer and receive support, and be introduced to useful contacts. Some midwives may consider 'networking' will produce for them a conflict of interest because of the competitive nature of NHS Trusts. On the contrary, 'networking' usually improves personal confidence and thus creates a healthy desire for new ideas and to perform effectively at work.

Personal suggestions for midwifery managers

The following tips are taken from *Business Now* (1994) and are reproduced for midwifery managers to use when they feel others are 'piling on the pressure':

- When you start to feel stressed, give yourself fifteen minutes to plan your day. List everything you want to achieve, and estimate how long it will take you.

- If you have more work than there are hours in the day, something's got to give. You may be able to defer work or delegate.

- If certain jobs aren't going to get done, say so to whoever is affected. Tell them the reason, that you have been prioritizing, and when their work will be done.

- Schedule the rest of your day. Build in two minutes every hour for a brief relaxation exercise. This will mean you will work more effectively for the other 58 minutes or so.

- Be realistic - this is vital. If you know a job always take one hour, schedule one hour, despite the fact that you feel you should be working faster.

- Ask your secretary to reduce possible interruptions by informing relevant colleagues and staff that you are working on special projects and are busy.

- Adopt a positive attitude. Instead of thinking - 'how am I going to get through' tell yourself 'I can do it - and will feel great when I have done it'.

Violence in the workplace

'I have nothing new to teach the world. Truth and non-violence are as old as the hills.' (M. K. Gandhi, 1927).

Violence and aggression to professionals and people involved with the public is unfortunately on the increase. In some ways this is not completely surprising, especially as those who work in the National Health Service are involved with people who frequently feel anxious, vulnerable, very stressed and sometimes aggrieved. It is also a fact that, no matter how careful or thoughtful a member of staff may be, occasionally if someone decides to concentrate and direct their anger on them, whether expressed verbally or physically, it is not strictly their fault. The fatal stabbing attacks on two health workers, first a young occupational therapist in September 1993 and then a nursing sister whilst working in Intensive Care in June 1995, show how vulnerable health service staff are as they go about their work.

Although violence should not be condoned, equally staff have a right to be safe whilst at work, and should not be assaulted in any way whilst caring for others. The whole aspect of childbirth is extremely emotive and therefore midwives are particularly exposed to violence in one way or other, especially when working in such areas as the labour suite and in the community. Other domains such as the antenatal clinic, the neonatal unit and the postnatal wards can be also be hazardous, especially if expectations of the pregnancy or childbirth have not been met and anxious relatives are involved. Also there can be the problems associated with security, with staff working in hospitals which are open 24 hours a day, where there are several entrances into a hospital, and the grounds are large and often poorly lit. More frequently the perpetrator of violence in these situations is not known to the member of staff.

Ensuring safety at work is the employer's responsibility, and those in management positions must make every effort to safeguard and protect their staff. It therefore rests with midwifery managers and midwifery sisters to guarantee that up-to-date procedures are in place, which are clearly understood and carried out. According to 'The National Health Service (Amendment) Act - 1987' - Health and Safety at Work Act - employers must safeguard, as far as is reasonably practicable, the health, safety and welfare of the people who work for them, and this covers staff who face predictable risk of verbal and physical abuse.

It therefore follows that managers have a responsibility to their staff to create an environment which is safe and healthy. To be able to do this managers must have knowledge about violence and aggression, why it occurs, how to deal with violent incidents and the after-effects of a violent incident. Although staff have a duty to take 'reasonable care' to avoid injury to themselves, safety policies must be in place to support them. Also, it is worth remembering that staff exercising 'self defence' to protect themselves must operate within the law. Additionally midwives have extra professional responsibilities imposed upon them by their registration body the UKCC for Nursing, Midwifery and Health Visiting, which is accountable for setting and maintaining professional standards.

The characteristics of aggression

According to Robertson (1993) there are two types of aggression:

- Angry aggression - which is the most common. This involves emotional arousal through displacement (when a person takes their anger out on other people) and transference (which is when the aggression experienced by a person has been transferred to them from someone else).

- Instrumental aggression - less common, but can be extremely frightening. It is a cold and calculating attempt by a person, apparently without conscience, to gain maximum benefit for themselves whilst carrying out the aggression.

Robertson gives the most popular theories connected with violence and aggression as:

Instinct theories

These are mainly based on Sigmund Freud's work. These assert that aggression is a 'natural instinct' in all of us. The weakness of these theories is that the exact nature of 'aggressive instinct' remains unclear. Questions such as 'why are some people more aggressive than others?', 'why do some people react with violence when others are able to "shrug off" their anger?' and 'why do some people appear not to react at all?' are not answered at all.

Frustration theory

This has emerged due to the 'shortcomings' of the instinct theories, in an attempt to redress the imbalance. Fundamentally this theory maintains that frustration is always a cause of aggression, and that aggression is always a result of frustration. Still this fails to explain why not all frustration leads to aggression.

Social learning theory

This sustains the argument that aggression is learnt in a social context. This theory claims that aggressive behaviour is not hereditary but is learnt and expressed aggressive feelings and behaviour are learnt by direct reward. It therefore follows that aggression is governed and controlled by human thought processes i.e. cognitive processes - the influence of family, friends and peers and 'distance modelling' - the influence of the media, films and television.

Verbal assault

Verbal assault is violence. The difficulty that arises for midwives with this type of assault is that the offender may be the mother for whom they are caring, and the verbal abuse may be associated with pain and distress which the mother is experiencing, especially during labour. Situations vary, and the setting and the extent to which the midwife can respond as a professional must be taken into consideration. More usually the perpetrator is a close relative of the mother, an anxious husband or partner and in this situation the midwife will have to decide how much verbal abuse she is prepared to tolerate. Also the midwife needs to be confident that the action being taken is supported by her employer. Failure to handle verbal abuse properly can quickly escalate into aggression.

Verbal assault occurring at work can make midwives feel unsafe and the midwifery manager has a responsibility to try to alleviate these feelings. The production of guidelines, agreed and written in conjunction with the staff, will provide accepted techniques on how verbal assault can be dealt with. The following techniques should be included:

Control of breathing
How the member of staff can concentrate on their own breathing and not so sharply on what is going on around them. Breathing in a steady and smooth way will reduce the immediate debilitating effect of fear - the panic which causes one to 'freeze' and will allow time to decide on what course of action to take in defence.

Personal behaviour
* speak in a lowered voice
* sit down when speaking
* say nothing.

Action
Possibilities include:
* enquire what is wrong and try to rationalize with the person
* ask the person to stop being so abusive
* leave the room
* call (by telephone if available) and get a colleague to join in
* do nothing.

Reporting the incident
- verbally
- completion of accident or incident form
- record keeping.

When violence is threatened

Sometimes the offender will use intimidating language and behave in a threatening manner to frighten a member of staff, or use this type of behaviour as a forerunner to actual physical assault. Such behaviour includes:

- being pinned against the wall
- being told 'you' cannot leave the room
- hands being placed around the throat
- picking up a weapon - an ashtray, chair, office equipment etc.

Staff have a right to defend and protect themselves in this situation. It is a myth that because midwives work in a professional capacity they should not be able to do so. Self-defence is referred to in Section 3 of 'The Criminal Law Act' (1967) which permits the 'use of reasonable force in the act of defending yourself.' Rogers and Salvage (1988) believe, however, that self-defence should only be used as a last resort if the health professional is unable to get help or to escape. Additional techniques on how to deal with threatening situations should also be included in the guidelines as follows:

Action
- if possible remove oneself from the situation
- make an excuse to leave the room
- suggest a further meeting at another time - possibly with someone else present.

Physical attack or assault

In this situation the aggressor has made a decision to physically control or hurt another person - in this case the member of staff. This type of violent behaviour can vary widely and can include:

- grasping and pulling hair
- wrenching and twisting the wrists
- grabbing the throat
- pinning the person to the floor
- attacking with weapons

How the member of staff responds is a question of degree. Whether to run away, or protect and preserve their 'own-person' is dependent on the situation but the following action should be taken:

- do everything within one's power to remove oneself from the situation as quickly as possible

- if the staff member feels she or he has to stay to protect someone else, or a group of people, it is important that an attempt is made to work out in their mind what they expect to achieve by staying, and how they are going to do it.

Immediately following the incident

A medical examination should take place. A visit to the Accident and Emergency Department is necessary if serious injuries have been sustained, or to the Occupational Health Department or to their own GP.

Completing a written report

Contemporaneous records must be made, which include making a note of everything that led up to the incident, what happened during the incident and immediately following it. Everyone involved in the situation must be included in the report, what part they played and how or what they contributed to the event and the final outcome.

Subsequent to a violent incident

A supporting relationship between the midwifery manager and member of staff who experiences a violent incident is crucial. As soon as possible after the event opportunity should be given for discussion and examination of feelings. Some staff may be afraid they could loose their job following such an incident. In fact there are no victors as far as violence is concerned. Usually the staff-member feels apprehensive and anxious and in need of help and support at work. The manager must be sensitive to future arrangements, by respecting the person's feelings and not putting undue pressure on her i.e. when planning a return to work, possibly in the same work environment. Often professional counselling is recommended, as staff who experience violence at work commonly suffer after-effects that can be very long-term. Also, according to Lamplugh (1988) legal advice should normally be available from a solicitor when necessary, and this should now be covered in the Trust's Assault Risk Policy.

After-effects of violence can vary, but can be exhausting and consume much of a person's time and energy. They include:

- constant fretting over what happened
- fear and doubt about the events that led up to the incident and whether it could have been avoided or prevented
- loss of confidence and self-worth.

Support from the midwifery manager is about honesty and caring about what happens to their staff. It's about letting someone else share an experience, learning more about the situation and passing information on to other staff for their benefit. Without managerial support, counselling where appropriate and help work-colleagues, the chances of a person getting over the effects of severe violence and aggression are quite remote.

At the same time the midwifery manager should inform senior managers - the Clinical Director, directors of the NHS Trust Board - of what has happened, what is being done, and if there are any changes in policy and why. In this way a culture of cooperation will be developed.

Monitoring violence to staff

Most NHS Trusts monitor violence to staff, including verbal abuse, and will have a formal reporting system to find out:

- where incidents occur
- how often
- if any time of the day or night presents more of a problem
- whether the incident could have been prevented i.e. with improved security, lighting etc.

Midwifery managers, by publicising and sharing their own 'monitoring findings of notified violence' with their staff will increase peoples awareness about the problem. More importantly this will encourage individual members to report incidents, however small, so that safety in the workplace can continue to be improved.

Midwives working in the community

The legal rights and responsibilities of community midwives are included in the same legislation which covers midwives working in the hospital environment. As community midwives also work in non NHS premises, mainly travel alone in their car and carry out home visits, they are particularly vulnerable in these situations. Also community midwives are more likely to be on their own during the early hours of the morning, have to find house and street locations, and are targets for abuse because of drugs and equipment they carry. Sometimes these risk issues can cause difficulties with motor insurance cover.

Effective procedures to reduce the risk of violence to community midwives should include:

- calling upon 'high risk families' in pairs.
- administrating and monitoring night calls for community midwives through Labour suite or another ward in the maternity unit.
- notifying the midwifery manager/office or colleagues when potential 'at risk' home visits are to be carried out.
- after darkness visiting in pairs, or having an arrangement where the community midwife informs the hospital of the time she is leaving for a home visit, where she is going, and informing them when she returns to her own home again.
- holding clinics instead of home visits in isolated and dangerous areas.

- using alarms, two-way radios or portable telephones.
- getting the midwife to use her own professional judgement when assessing the mother and baby and the home situation, especially when the mother refuses to be visited during the statutory period of visiting. By informing her Supervisor of Midwives and writing a report on these situations, the problem can be shared and appropriate action taken.
- avoiding evening meetings.

Recently, as reported by Betty (1995) courses in 'defensive driving' are providing community staff with more ideas on how to protect themselves. Major elements of a one day course were devoted to personal security, defensive driving skills - accompanied by an instructor, low speed manoeuvring and parking. Although some staff were suspicious of the motives for the training at first, post-course evaluation showed high levels of satisfaction.

Creating a 'healthy awareness' about violence at work

Guidelines for dealing with violence in the workplace are necessary, but they can only give suggestions and directions on what could happen, and how things can be handled in a particular situation. In order to develop a more meaningful and shared understanding about violence and aggression, these subjects need be discussed openly amongst the staff.

The responsibility for creating a 'healthy awareness' about violence rests with the midwifery manager and the midwifery sisters in the wards, departments and community. Agenda items for formal meetings should include violence and aggression, and staff should be encouraged to discuss these subjects openly during informal gatherings. In this way a mutual understanding will be built up of what is considered threatening and unacceptable behaviour. Although opinions will vary at first, at least there will be an agreement, especially amongst those practising at the 'front line of care', on what is threatening and unacceptable behaviour, so there will be no confusion about when they can support each other and when not to get involved.

Training workshops
On how to manage aggression

Training is essential, and can be provided externally or internally, but is better given 'in-house' so staff and managers can benefit from the shared learning experience. Venues can vary but by using rooms in the maternity unit, the full range of the maternity services can be covered - including aspects of the community. Training in individual wards and departments for smaller groups of staff with their midwifery sister, is ideal for team building and teamworking.

Topics may include:
- Cause and process of aggression, conflict and violence
- The nature of the professional and caring relationship of the midwife, the mother and her family

- The role of communication and support from others in creating and solving conflict
- Practical ways of responding, or not responding, to violence
- The differences between aggression, conflict and violence and the way they can exhibit in the work environment in both the hospital and community settings
- Reporting procedures - keeping records, completing the incident form and writing reports
- Breathing and relaxation techniques
- Practical self defence techniques.

The practical sessions are good for demonstrating through experiential learning, the difficulty of physical action combined with concentration, and allow staff the experience of facing a threat of violence from another person in a safe environment. Robertson (1993) found the use of an 'air-filled bag' allowed course-members the opportunity to strike. Hitting an inanimate object was quite difficult for many of the participants and this underlined the inhibitions that many people have about physical action, particularly against a client or their close relative, even if they are dangerous or otherwise.

Additional management responsibilities in the prevention and reduction of violent incidents to staff

Security of buildings
- security systems and equipment
- video monitoring at the entrance to the Maternity Unit
- controlled video or audio monitoring at the entrance to each ward and department, so that staff can speak with, and identify visitors to the ward prior to allowing them to enter
- alarm systems connected to 'switchboard' or a security control desk
- keeping only one central entrance open at night
- improving lighting in corridors and hospital grounds at night
- installing secure locks on doors and windows, especially where minimal staff work during unsocial hours
- secure car parking.

Personal security of staff
- alarm buttons in wards and departments which are wired to 'ring' in adjoining wards or departments: 'switchboard' or security control desk.
- personal alarms and/or portable telephones for community midwives.

Staffing
- wherever possible community midwives to work in 'pairs' when going out during hours of darkness i.e. to a home confinement or Parent Education classes
- ensure adequate security personnel patrol the hospital buildings and grounds. These must be in proportion to the size of the hospital.

Work environment

- use appointment systems in antenatal clinic and community clinics to avoid long waits, reduce frustration and prevent aggression
- medical and midwifery staff to be available and ready to commence clinic appointments on time
- 'notices' regarding the length of waiting time in antenatal clinics to give the mother some idea of the time she may have to wait
- provide a 'homely environment' to encourage relaxation
- locate staff changing rooms in a busy part of the hospital to avoid isolation, especially during unsocial hours.

With demands increasing for the provision of a high quality maternity service, the general public expect care during pregnancy and childbirth to be given proficiently, and their baby to be born alive and healthy. When things don't go as expected, frustration occurs and it is usually the midwives at the front-line of care who have to deal with dissatisfied customers and or their relatives.

It is well recognized that staff at the front line need to be increasingly aware of situations that are potentially violent, and know how to deal with them. Sound procedures, support and understanding from the midwifery manager are crucial.

Summary

Creating a healthy and safe work environment is the aim of every NHS employer and is bound in law. Employers have a responsibility to safeguard the health, safety and welfare of staff as is reasonably practical. Despite these safeguards stressors can still develop in the workplace, and are often associated with the type of work staff do.

Baby snatching

The kidnapping of three babies from Maternity Units in the past five years has dismayed the public. Each time the baby snatcher has been a woman, who has kidnapped for her own selfish needs and not for maternal desire. Mothers and midwives are traumatised following a baby snatch. The midwifery manager's monitoring and supportive role is essential for resolving the situation objectively and preventing long term after effects.

Action to deter baby snatchers is necessary. Guidelines can ensure Maternity Units remain safe without adopting a 'fortress mentality'.

Complaints

Nobody likes complaints. This is especially so when the complaint is made against the midwife and her professional practice. Mothers and their families expect high standards of care, and since the *Patients Charter* (1991) the number of complaints has risen sharply.

The main reasons for complaints include inadequate care and treatment, wrong attitude of staff and poor communication. Complaints affect mothers, midwives and managers in different ways.

Complaints must be handled sensitively, investigated speedily and resolved satisfactorily. Unfortunately many midwives experience extreme stress during complaint investigations, and even if exonerated can suffer long term effects.

The new NHS complaints procedure, due to be implemented in April 1996, promises to be a fairer arrangement for mothers and midwives, with its aim for a 'single, simple and speedier' system.

Stress at work

Stress can be a positive force, but is usually associated with negativity. Negative stress is a major occupational hazard and accounts for high levels of absenteeism in the NHS. Stress presents itself in various ways and usually involves unpleasant under-or-over stimulation which can lead to ill health. Stress can be caused by personal problems or work induced factors. 'Burnout', a manifestation of stress, includes negative self concepts and negative attitudes to work. One person experiencing 'burnout' can lower the morale in the workplace.

Stress can be dealt with positively and individuals can reduce their stress levels by developing their own techniques. Midwifery managers can reduce work-induced stress through sound organizational management.

Violence

Violence and aggression to those involved with the public is increasing. NHS workers are vulnerable because they deal with people who frequently feel anxious. Childbirth is emotive and midwives are exceptionally exposed when things go wrong. Violence from someone unknown can also occur in health service premises and employers have a responsibility to ensure 24 hour safety.

Understanding aggression is important and how to manage situations of verbal and physical assault. Reporting violence is essential and also the supporting role of the midwifery manager.

Midwives in the community are vulnerable to violence because they travel alone and go out at night. Effective procedures can help prevent the risks to the community midwives.

Creating a healthy awareness about violence can be achieved through discussion, education and training. Managers have a responsibility for preventing, reducing and monitoring violent incidents.

CHAPTER SEVEN

Effective Communication

'Communication is like a piece of driftwood on a sea of conflicting currents.
Sometimes the shore will be littered with debris,
sometimes again it will be bare.

The amount and direction of movement is not aimless or indirectional
but is a response to all the forces - winds, tides, and currents - which
come into play.' (Jay M. Jackson)

Communication is the most important skill in management. Everything a manager does involves communication. In fact the ability to communicate is central to life itself. A manager who cannot communicate cannot manage people, and people are what make organizations work.

Effective communication is the key to success in any organization, whether it is face to face, in writing, over the telephone or during presentations. Yet, according to Cooper (1994) communication in the National Health Service is poor, and probably at its lowest point ever. He attributes this to senior staff still not understanding the importance of effective communication with those at the 'practical level', which in turn can effect their performance and standards of patient care. In April 1994, an Audit Commission Report strongly recommended NHS Trusts improve the quality of information they give to their nursing staff, after more than half of hospital and community staff they questioned said they felt they were not well informed by management about what their Trust was doing. Managers must set good examples in communication, but sometimes there is a tendency to use management 'jargon', which does not help others to understand.

Midwives certainly know the importance of good communication, and during the past five years there has been great emphasis on how they can develop and improve their interpersonal skills. Today, communication is included in the curriculum of midwifery pre registration diploma and degree courses and through continuing and in-service education. Also there is a vast amount of literature on the subject in the midwifery and nursing press. But have midwives improved their communication skills? Magill-Cuerden (1992) points out that the midwife's role is not an easy one, especially when 'treading a line' between enabling and supporting women with their needs and choices, and meeting the policies and guidelines produced by the Maternity Services Unit.

Changing Childbirth (1993) advocates women centred care, so midwives more than ever before will be required to communicate effectively to ensure each mother's care is planned according to her specific needs and preferences. Imparting knowledge through open communication will form the basis on which the mother will make her 'informed choices', but much more than this will be the special relationship that develops between the mother and the midwife. This can only come about through sensitive two way communication.

For the midwifery manager the challenge is two-fold. Firstly, self directed to achieve effective communication skills as a manager and leader, and secondly, facilitating midwives and other maternity workers in maternity care to communicate effectively with mothers and their families, their managers, colleagues and other health professionals.

Defining communication

'Man' is the only animal who can:

- organize and reorganize his vocabulary to express feelings, thoughts, needs and emotions in countless situations
- translate verbal messages into written messages
- express himself in movement and gesture.

Although human beings communicate all their lives, it is not a case where practice makes perfect, so often communications break down.

Many definitions exist which include:

'all that occurs between two or more minds' (Shannon and Weaver in La Monica, 1994)

'interchange of thought or information to bring about a mutual understanding' (American Society of Training Directors)

Communication is therefore a human-to-human activity which always involves a transmitter or sender and a recipient or receiver (Fig. 7.1).

- it involves using the sense organs, mainly hearing and sight, the emotions, thought and the interpretation of information
- it cannot be carried out in isolation
- if the person being communicated with does not understand or want to communicate, then there is no communication
- the end result of communication is a change in both the sender and the receiver
- communication is based on shared experience only

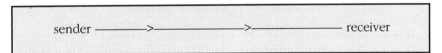

sender ———>———————>————— receiver

Fig. 7.1: Sender transmits to receiver

The effect of communication will depend upon:

- Prior feelings: attitudes, opinions and prejudices that the participants have towards each other, their perceptions and how they view each other
- Pre existing expectations and motives of the persons communicating.
- What is being communicated: the content, clarity and message, and whether it is agreeable, understood, accepted or rejected.

The process of communication

The communication process involves five essential steps (Fig. 7.2):

1.   Idea. The sender has an idea and wants to communicate this to another person. The idea has come about as a result of thinking and using the thought processes.

2.   Encode. Once the sender has the idea clearly in mind this has to be encoded, and the suitable language selected. Usually this is by speech or in writing. When face to face communication is the method of choice, non-verbal body language will need to be carefully thought about as well as the verbal language.

3.   Transmit. The message is transmitted by the sender by the chosen method, either by speech or in writing.

4.   Decode. The receiver needs to be 'in tune' with the sender to receive the message, and decode it from the language of the sender to their own language.

5   Idea. The receiver forms an idea from the decoded message and acts in response. This may be to:

- send another idea back to the sender
- perform a task or activity as a direct result of the message
- remember the information for use later
- decide not to do anything with it.

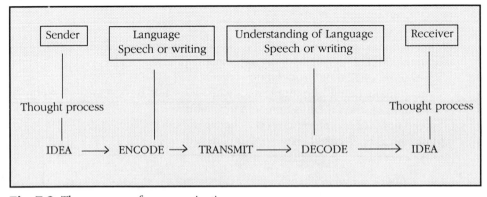

Fig. 7.2: The process of communication

Whatever response the receiver decides upon is known as 'feedback' to the sender. If the receiver decides to communicate an idea back in reply to the sender then the five steps in the communication process start again (Fig. 7.3). This cycle will continue until communication stops.

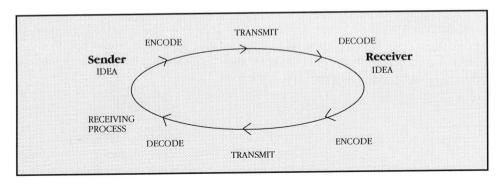

Fig. 7.3: The cycle of communication

In order for the sender to evaluate feedback an assessment needs to be made on whether the message has been perceived as intended by the receiver. This will be facilitated through listening and watching. The objective of communication is that there is a similar understanding between the sender's intended message and the recipient's perceived message. Unfortunately this can go terribly wrong.

Barriers to successful communication

The fundamental problem in communication is that the meaning which is actually received may not be what the sender intended. The sender and the receiver are two different people, with different personalities, occupying different lives and valuing different things. It is not surprising that a number of things can happen to distort the intended message, as it passes through a number of stages (Fig. 7.4).

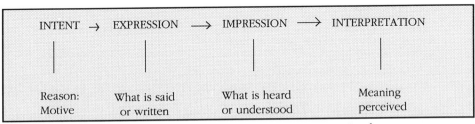

Fig. 7.4: The stages involved from intended message to perceived message.

Reasons why communication breaks down

THE RECEIVER HEARS ONLY WHAT SHE OR HE WANTS TO HEAR

This may be as a result of past experience and background, so that the message is interpreted to fit in with the receiver's expectations. This includes stereotyping, by which the receiver attributes the same characteristics to a particular group of people e.g. managers, midwives, ethnic groups, religious denomination and so on.

In these circumstances the attitude of the receiver will influence their perception of what the person is saying, or is not saying. Sometimes the receiver has what is described as 'emotional noise in the head' which is so loud and distorted that communication may not even take place.

NOT LISTENING

The receiver does not pay attention to what is being said, or is thinking about other things and misses the point. The receiver may be distracted by outside or internal noise, other activities going on at the same time, or simply just not listening.

STATUS

There is no doubt status and power influence communication. A midwifery manager who resorts to an autocratic approach will inhibit feedback and upward-communication. A member of staff who has anxieties about management may restrict communication with the boss, even though the manager is communicating well and using a participative style of communication. Sometimes the subordinate in this situation may give the midwifery manager information which she thinks the manager wants to hear, and not what they 'fear' the manager should not know.

The possibility that a manager may respond with sarcasm or be off-hand, may also deter staff from making an approach. This can also arise from the manager's perspective. A manager may select certain behaviours to protect her status by keeping a distance and avoiding any challenges and confrontations from below.

IGNORING INFORMATION THAT CONFLICTS WITH WHAT WE ALREADY KNOW

When there is a resistance to change there is a tendency to reject a new idea, especially if it conflicts with what we already believe. Through 'filtering' the information there is a inclination to accept that which agrees with our beliefs and ignore, or even eliminate, anything that conflicts with them.

When communication is consistent with the beliefs of a person the recipient will:

* respond more readily to what is being said
* seek more information
* accept the information as valuable
* remember what is heard
* store accurately in the memory

When communication is inconsistent with the beliefs of a person the recipient will:

* respond reluctantly
* not seek additional information
* reject the validity of the information
* quickly forget
* store distorted information in the memory.

THE WAY WE 'SEE' OTHERS

There is a tendency to see people either as positive or negative and not as neutral and this can influence the way the receiver perceives the sender's message. This sometimes results in what Tyes (1982) calls the 'Halo Effect', when someone is admired to such a degree that the receiver fails to see their weaknesses. This may be someone in a senior position and their view is accepted at 'face value' because of this. On the other hand, if someone is disliked so much the receiver will not hear anything good they say, or they may attach 'uncharitable rationalisation to such communications'.

THE USE OF LANGUAGE AND TECHNICAL TERMS OR JARGON

Semantic difficulties will occur if words that mean different things to different people, are used to transmit the idea, such as plant or theatre.

Professional jargon, the use of abbreviations and technical language, whilst having a meaning to a particular group of people e.g. managers, midwives, doctors, computer technicians are unhelpful when used to people outside the specific group.

EMOTIONS

Different emotions will effect communications in distinct ways. If a person is:

*   angry - there is an inclination to attach blame and hurt in most communications
*   depressed - everything is seen negatively and maybe distorted, which is reflected in communications
*   elated - being 'on a high' can result in criticisms and problems being ignored or not even recognized
*   fear, anxiety and insecurity - tend to cause incorrect interpretation of messages, and completely innocent or harmless communications can be seen as threatening.

Walton (1988) considers the National Health Service is an organization 'cradled in anxiety' because of the tasks it is asked to perform and the setting in which staff work. He believes that people who work in the health service will be emotionally and personally affected by the jobs they do and the status of people around them. Consequently, it is necessary to adjust the style of communication to the way others are observed to be behaving and help them to understand.

NON VERBAL SIGNALS AND BODY LANGUAGE

Even when the sender is speaking clearly and using the correct language to help the receiver, certain non verbal signals can effect the communication, such as:

*   posture, mannerisms, standing or sitting, facial expression, no eye-to eye contact, pointing etc.
*   non verbal clues tell a lot about both the sender and receiver, and provide valuable information when assessing feedback.

Why does communication matter?

A breakdown or a failure in communication can be extremely costly. The midwifery manager to do her job must get work done through others, by motivating them to accomplish goals, and must be able to communicate effectively. This also applies to midwifery sisters in their leadership and management roles, and other midwives performing delegated management responsibilities. According to La Monica (1994) good communication is the 'bridge' on which teamwork rests, and teamwork results in:

- high quality
- decreased costs
- high employee morale

Davies and Newstrom (La Monica, 1994) identified an equation to define the purpose of communication as:

the skill to work + the will to work = communication.

The purposes of communication are many, and are not usually used in isolation but with each other. The main reasons for the midwifery manager are:

- to get an understanding throughout the Maternity Services and the NHS Trust at all levels - downwards, upwards and across
- to influence another person's behaviour or the behaviour of a group
- to foster a willingness in others
- to achieve goals - personal and for the Maternity Services
- to achieve change
- to relate to others and express feelings
- to teach, instruct and learn new knowledge, skills and experiences
- to reduce tension and resolve conflict.

If midwives and maternity services staff are to give of their best they need to feel valued, intrinsically motivated and part of the team. When communications are inferior, poor performance and low morale will result. If this happens staff will develop distorted views of what others are doing and hostility is likely to result. This in turn could develop into open conflict, or the repression of ill-feelings. According to Tyes (1982) 'breakdowns in communication may foster hostility and hostility interferes with communication'.

The successful midwifery manager will use sound communication processes to transmit accurate and effective information to staff and work colleagues and to obtain and assimilate information to achieve the Maternity Services goals.

Types of communication

Fundamentally communications can be classified into:

- verbal or oral - frequently supported by non verbal
- written and graphic
- both written and oral

Also people can communicate images and impressions through the way they dress, behave and present themselves.

Verbal

The spoken word will take up the majority of the midwifery manager's time, whether this is face to face or over the telephone.

FACE TO FACE COMMUNICATION

Although verbal communication is the most frequently used method of communication it is not a particularly efficient method because of the many distortions that may arise (see barriers to communication).

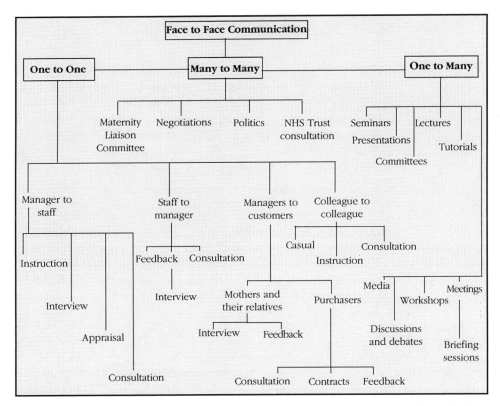

Fig 7.5: Showing the extensive range of face to face communication that the midwifery manager is likely to be involved in.

If a message can be distorted between two individuals, then not surprisingly a message can be distorted many times over during open meetings with staff, other managers, customers, purchasers of Maternity Services and user groups.

Effective verbal communication requires the following skills:

- Sound preparation - if thoughts are unclear so will the sentences that are spoken
- Thinking before speaking - sometimes the wrong interpretation can be given because just one word has a different significance
- Setting the scene - by giving an outline of what is under discussion. Sometimes it may be considered helpful to give some background information.
- Aiming for clarity in audibility and tone of voice - pronunciation is important and so is the speed of delivering the message. A monotonous voice can inhibit interest and affect understanding, and a long drawn out message can be a 'turn off' for the receiver
- Tuning into the world of the listener - by trying to understand the feelings and beliefs of the receiver. Listening 'between the lines' to what is not said as much as what is said. Listening with 'the third ear' attuned to understanding the unspoken meanings of words
- Seeking to establish eye to eye contact
- Reducing 'offputting' non verbal signals
- Observing for immediate reactions
- Encouraging feedback though discussion.

Nelson (1992) asserts that all business communication, which is now the 'world' of the midwifery manager, has an element of negotiated order about it. This means that a once the starting point has been agreed, communication will be one of proposition and response, defining and clarifying. As long as genuine opportunity is given for feedback, correction, reinforcement and comment, the clearer and more defined the communication will be.

USING THE TELEPHONE

This is a thoroughly modern method of communication, in an age where mobile phones are customary and telecommunications are becoming progressively more sophisticated. The telephone is one of the most powerful tools available in business today, and every call - incoming, outgoing or internal- will add to the success of the organization if practical techniques are used. For example, deciding the best time to use the telephone, and how much time to spend on the phone.

Communicating by telephone is verbal communication without the non verbal signals. Added to this could be the problem of 'silence'. This means the choice of words and what is actually being said, plus clarity and tone are all crucially important. Should there be any doubt about the receiver misinterpreting what has been said, it is wise to summarize before ending the call. This can then be followed up in writing, confirming the conversation and the result of the phone call.

The timing of a telephone call is also very important, so the receiver can give their full attention to what is being said. A good way of assuring the correct time is for the secretary to book a 'telephone meeting' for the midwifery manager, for five minutes or longer if required. This will allow for a period of uninterrupted discussions. When telephoning the wards, departments and midwives in the community, the midwifery manager should try to avoid busy times e.g. report handover. Likewise it is important to let staff know when the midwifery manager is accessible for incoming telephone calls, and the manager should make sure this time remains available.

When someone has phoned and it is not convenient, the secretary should tell them when to phone back, or when the midwifery manager will return their call. Remember, it may have taken a member of staff a lot of courage and effort to make that telephone call. When a manager promises to be available or to phone back it is only courteous to do so, as there is nothing more annoying than waiting for a call that doesn't come.

LISTENING

According to Cava (1991) we spend up to 80 per cent of our conscious hours using the communication skills of writing, reading, speaking and listening. Listening accounts for more than 50 per cent of this time, but most of us are not able to give close attention to what is being said for more than sixty seconds at a time.

Listening involves the ability to 'tune into people, the environment and the meaning of messages that are spoken and unspoken' (La Monica, 1994). Unfortunately most of us do not 'actively listen' to what others are saying. We hear but so often do not perceive the message which the sender intended. Davis and Newstrom (La Monica, 1994) have taken this concept further and assert that 'one hears with one's ears but listening occurs in the mind'. Skills in the art of listening willingly and attentively can be learned. and the advantages for midwifery managers and midwives cannot be ignored. When listening is 'active' messages will be received accurately and time will be saved. Better decision-making will also result.

Cava (1991) gives an interesting insight into the 'world of the speaker and listener'. She tells us the normal speaking-speed is 125-150 words per minute, rising to 160 words per minute for a person conducting a seminar. As for listening, we are capable of listening at the phenomenal speed of 750-1,200 words per minute. So why don't we hear what people tell us? Cava believes this is because we are bored and because there is not enough to keep the brain occupied at normal speeds of speech. To help improve listening skills she gives a number of hints, some of which are reproduced below:

- There must be motivation to want to improve. Without this it will be too much effort.
- Try to find an uninterrupted area in which to converse. Keeping your train of thought is difficult when there are obstructions to concentration.
- Try not to anticipate what the other person will say.
- Be mindful of your own biases and prejudices, so they don't unduly influence your listening.

- Pay careful attention to what is being said. Don't stop listening in order to plan a rebuttal to a particular point.
- Don't allow yourself to get too far ahead of the speaker by trying to understand things too soon.
- At intervals, try to paraphrase what people have been saying. Give them the opportunity to learn what you have heard them say.
- When you have difficulty determining the point of the speaker's remarks, say, 'Why are you telling me this?'
- Watch for key or buzz words if you find you've lost the train of the conversation. This happens particularly when the speaker is long-winded or has a tendency to ramble.

A good listener is someone who:

- lets another person finish what they are saying without interrupting
- shows they are paying attention by comfortable eye-to-eye contact, and not letting their eyes wander around the room
- asks questions if they are not sure
- remains open minded and ready to review their opinion
- pays attention to non verbal signals
- listens with the 'third ear' to what is not being said as much as what is being said.

Responding skills

To facilitate the communication process there are a number of skills that can be used. Frequently people need help to clarify what they are trying to say, and once this is recognized and accepted sensitive prompting can take place. Of course different responding skills will be required for different situations, but generally the skills can be used to enhance every day communication.

- Questioning: the use of open questions rather than closed - 'How did you feel...?' rather than 'Did you feel pleased?'

- Exploratory: 'Can you talk more about that...'

- Clarifying: 'Do you mean that...?' or 'I'm not sure I understand what you are saying'

- Empathic: 'It sounds as though you feel...'

- Interpreting: 'Are you really saying...'

- Supportive: 'It sounds as if it was really a success...'

- Reflective: by repeating statements in a sensitive reflective way.

- Silences: let them be for a while, do not feel uncomfortable with them.

- Non verbal communication: be aware of body language - posture, movement, facial expressions, eye contact etc.

Non verbal communication

Non verbal communication is the language of the body. This can be communicated powerfully through a person's behaviour, whether intentional or without knowing. The importance of posture, facial expression, eye contact and tone of the voice have already been recognized, all of which can intensify or reduce interactions between two or more people. Although non verbal communication usually accompanies oral communication, it can be significantly judged on its own.

Morris (1977) refers to 'nonverbal leakage' being the clues that give us away without our knowing. He says 'nonverbal leakage is the failure of the social mask'. So often we put on a happy face in public when in reality we feel nervous and tense, but generally our body posture gives away valuable clues of what we really feel. This is because a person is not always fully conscious of the degree of stiffness in their stance, or their slump and alertness. A person is even less aware of hand movements, and least aware of leg and foot movements. This is one of the reasons a manager may feel more comfortable behind a desk during an interview or a negotiation. Morris maintains 'whole-body lying' is difficult because we lack practice.

According to Cava (1991) being able to interpret non verbal signals is probably one of the best assets anyone can have. For midwifery managers and midwives to be good communicators first it is necessary to be aware of the non verbal signals, and secondly to have an understanding of what they mean. Cava has supplied some extremely useful examples of what non verbal language can tell us:

- Tapping fingers: the person is annoyed, impatient or anxious.
- Shifting weight from one foot to another: the person has been standing too long, or is impatient.
- Flushed face: the person is embarrassed, angry or hot, or has high blood pressure - other non verbal signs would have to be looked for to confirm which one it is.
- Slumped posture: the person is tired, relaxed or depressed.
- Avoidance of eye contact: the person is shy, or bored or may come from a culture that regards eye contact with those in positions of authority as disrespectful. This signal is often misinterpreted as a sign of shifty behaviour or lack of confidence, when the cause may be something quite different.
- Rapid or abrupt speech: the person is upset, worried, anxious or angry.
- Rise in voice pitch: in women - a sign that person is nervous or angry.
- Drop in voice pitch: in men - a sign that person is nervous or angry.
- Shrugging: the person is indifferent or doesn't know the answer.
- Forehead slapping: the person feels forgetful or stupid.
- Arms across the chest: the person feels defensive, physically cold or physically awkward.
- Nose scratching: the person is puzzled or dislikes something or the person's nose may be cold.
- Holding the hand up, palm outwards: the person is saying 'stop'.

Touch and 'whether to touch or not'

We often place a hand on the arm or shoulder of someone who is upset to show we understand and care. But, today sexual harassment in the workplace is receiving much more attention, and in consequence some people will avoid initiating any physical contact with work colleagues. Midwives know that touch can be therapeutic, but in the management situation it is also important to know when it is appropriate or not to use this form of non verbal communication.

Shaking hands with people

A firm handshake as a greeting or during a first meeting, indicates a high degree of self confidence. A handshake at the end of a meeting can mean a 'seal' of something that has been agreed, or indicates a person is loyal and can be trusted.

Leaning forwards or backwards

- Forwards - suggests a positive signal of interest
- Backwards - suggests a negative sign of disapproval or lack of interest.

Signals of 'power-hungry' people

These include deliberately interrupting, holding eye contact for longer than usual so the other person feels uncomfortable and looks away, hovering over others and watching them work.

Territorial invasions

People feel much more at ease when they are in their own territory. When a midwife comes to the midwifery manager's office the manager has the advantage, but when the midwifery manager visits the midwife in her own ward, the midwife has the advantage.

Consequently when a midwifery manager wants to speak to a midwife about something in general, it is better to go to the ward so the midwife feels less threatened. Alternatively they could meet in neutral 'territory', i.e. another room in the Maternity Unit. For a more serious problem it would be usual for the midwifery manager to ask the midwife to come to her office.

How to watch and reach people

McCormack (1985) has produced a seven step plan for what he calls 'learning to read people'. Although he admits there is no agreed number of steps to take and accepts that learning to read people cannot be taught in the classroom, he believes that by following a few basic fundamentals a person can open up their senses and be more receptive to others. This plan is adapted as follows:

Listen aggressively

Listen to not only what someone is saying, but how they are saying it. People will tell you more than they mean to. Keep pausing - a slight silence will tend to make them tell you more.

Observe aggressively

Watch posture, body language and gestures and 'hear' the statement someone may be making by the way they dress.

Talk less

You will automatically learn more, hear more, see more and make fewer blunders. Ask questions, but don't begin to answer them yourself.

Take a second look at first impressions

Only go with first impressions after you have carefully scrutinized them. Some 'thinking out' has to take place between your initial impression and your acceptance.

Take time to use what you've learned

If you are about to enter a discussion or make a phone-call or a presentation, take a moment to think about what you know and what you want to achieve. From what you know about the other person you should be able to work out what to say or do in order to get it.

Be discreet

Discretion is the better part of reading people. If you let them know what you know, you will blow away any chance of using your own insight effectively. You don't owe anyone an insight into yourself for every insight you have into them.

Be detached

If you can force yourself to step back from a situation that is heating up, your powers of observation will automatically increase. When another person gets heated they are more revealing than at almost any other time. Acting rather than reacting allows you to use what you have learnt. Reacting makes you less observant, and you reveal as much about yourself.

Writing skills

When choosing which method of communication to use it is necessary to first identify what message you want to send, its purpose and to whom it is intended.

A manager who wants to guarantee as many staff as possible are informed about something, will usually find it easier and more effective to communicate in writing.

However, Pearson and Thomas (1991) advise managers to avoid writing whenever possible and to use the telephone or internal memos instead. They recommend it is best to agree standard 'paragraphs' and letters for the secretary, so she can write routine letters and memos. With the advent of more sophisticated technology and internal computer systems, messages can more readily be relayed between offices, wards, departments and hospitals. This adds greatly to the speed of sending a message and getting a response, providing the receiver regularly switches into their 'electronic mail'.

There are numerous methods of communication by writing, which include:

- letters: circulars, memoranda
- notices: press releases
- agendas: minutes, notes of meetings
- leaflets: booklets
- handbooks: manuals
- questionnaires: reports
- charts: statistics, tables, flow charts.

With the written word there is little opportunity to clarify what has been written, and this is especially concerning if there is any ambiguity. The written word is in 'black and white', and will be a permanent record unless someone decides to discard it. Therefore before putting words on paper, or into the electronic message system, the successful midwifery manager will need to spend time on planning. Thinking carefully about the purpose of writing, who is going to read it, determining what will be included and what presentation to use.

'Ten Principles for Clear Writing' have been produced by Gunning (1968) and provide some of the best advice on how to write effectively. These are offered as follows:

1. Keep sentences short. Reading becomes difficult when sentences average more than twenty words. Sentences in the 'Reader's Digest' average seventeen words, much business writing exceeds twenty five words per sentence.

2. Prefer the simple to complex in sentence structure and in choice of words e.g. 'try to find out' rather than 'endeavour to ascertain'.

3. Prefer the familiar word to the far-fetched:
    - 'to use' rather than 'to utilize'
    - 'to keep apart' rather than 'to estrange'
    - 'to make widespread' rather than 'to promulgate'.

4. Avoid unnecessary words e.g. 'in connection with the position that has arisen with regard to…'

5. Put action into verbs e.g. 'you will see by reading' rather than 'it will be observed from the perusal of…'

6. Write the way you talk - not in stuffy business jargon.

7. Use terms your reader can picture. Abstract words make writing dull and obscure. Prefer the short, concrete words that stand for things you can see and touch e.g. 'her face was red' - 'his hands were cold'.

8. Tie in with your reader's experience. Your reader will receive your new ideas better if you link it with one of his or her ideas.

9. Make full use of variety. Avoid stilted, well-worn patterns of writing.

10. Write to express - not to impress. Don't show off with complexity. The writer who makes the best impression is the one who can express complex ideas simply.

Report writing

Reports and proposals are essential tools for midwifery managers. They simplify and clarify, and have a strong impact on the decision-making process. Equally they reflect the quality of the work being reported on, and the quality of the author.

> 'A report is a presentation of facts and findings, usually as a basis for recommendations; written for a specific readership and probably intended to be kept as a record' (PA International Management Consultants Ltd).

When writing a report it is sometimes easy for the midwifery manager to think that her report will be a major event in a reader's day, especially if the report is of particular importance and interest to her. In reality, other people are usually too busy to read the report. Senior managers tend to be inundated with reports, statistics and consultation documents. The success of any report is in its 'easily absorbed information' - just sufficient to keep the reader interested and come to a decision.

For effective report writing the following recommendations apply:

1. Define the major aim of the report - why is the report being written?

2. Identify:
    - who the reader(s) will be
    - what do they already know?
    - will they accept new ideas?
    - what are their expectations?

3. Set objectives - clarify what 'you' want the reader to consider and do after reading

4. Select material - include only the essential and discard the irrelevant

5. Structure of report:
    i)   Title page - with title, date, author's name and position - keep the page simple and uncluttered

ii)   Executive summary - write this in a stimulating way to attract the interest of the readers, and to give the gist of the report

iii)   Contents page - list sections and appendices, and give page numbers

iv)   Introduction
   - give the background to the report
   - explain why the report is justified
   - include the objective or objectives

v)   Body of the report - include the details, facts and findings and what information can be deduced from the findings

vi)   Conclusion
   - tease out the main points and draw them together
   - give a 'considered judgement'

vii)   Recommendations
   - set out any recommendations as a result of the findings
   - relate the recommendations clearly to the previous and current situation and then give the benefits for change

viii)   Appendices
   - give 'back-up' information i.e. graphs; tables, etc.
   - provide more detailed information which some readers may require

ix)   References
   - provide these when articles and books have been consulted for the report
   - provide for a suggested 'further reading' list

x)   Glossary
   - this is especially helpful for readers who are not familiar with medical and professional terms

6.   Layout and distribution of the report:
   - set the report out in a stylish manner
   - use wide margins, space out paragraphs and use sub-headings
   - type on one side of the paper only
   - number pages

   Decide how many copies for:
   - the principal readers
   - those on the distribution list
   - to be sent for interest and information only.

7.   Presentation of the report:
   - this can be by formal or informal presentation
   - decide your audience
   - establish the aims of the presentation and what to include
   - structure your presentation with an introduction, main body and conclusion
   - use visual aids
   - encourage discussion
   - evaluate feedback
   - decide upon future action.

Conducting effective meetings

Meetings enable groups of people, usually with a common interest, to come together to share ideas and experiences, and to make a contribution to the overall function and management of the organization. Whatever the size and composition of a meeting they have a common theme:

- they exist for a purpose
- they involve people communicating with each other
- they have a chairperson in control

Unfortunately some staff find meetings a waste of time, and others feel unable to participate because they find meetings intimidating. Smith (Pemberton, 1983) said poorly conducted meetings cost an organization dearly in terms of time, results and goodwill. Meetings should not become an end in themselves, and regular meetings should only be held when there is something worthwhile to discuss. Sometimes staff moan about attending routine meetings, possibly in the hope they might be discontinued. Meetings are an essential part of any organization - without meetings ideas would be lost and progress would cease. However meetings must be well planned and organized and have pertinent agenda items, so that staff can participate and contribute.

The role of the chairperson is crucial to any meeting. As midwifery managers and midwifery sisters take on more responsibilities in the flattened management structure they will find themselves more frequently chairing and conducting meetings. The role of the chairperson is to:

- plan, prepare and attend meetings regularly
- participate by asking questions, giving information, clarifying misunderstandings and correcting mistakes
- listen and analyse the meaning and relevance of what members say
- control the discussion during the meeting, and make it possible for all participants to contribute
- augment the contribution of ideas, experience and contributions of those attending
- effectively handle problem situations and difficult individuals
- extract the important and reject the irrelevancies
- ensure the purpose of the meeting is achieved within the allocated time
- liaise with the secretary to ensure a correct record is made for distribution.

Planning and preparation

A well planned meeting has much more chance of success than an unplanned one. This can be achieved by first defining the purpose of the meeting and writing down, in one or two sentences, why the meeting is necessary. This statement can then be read out at the beginning of the meeting. If no purpose can found then clearly there is no necessity for a meeting.

The agenda

Members of a meeting must know in advance what is going to be discussed.

*   the agenda will provide the topics for discussion to enable members to come prepared.
*   the agenda will give the time and date of the meeting, who is expected to be in attendance, the venue, and the expected length of the meeting.
*   the agenda should be circulated well in advance of the meeting - five days is preferable. Although, there may be occasions when the agenda is distributed with the previous minutes or notes. Relevant reports or written summaries should be circulated at the same time as the agenda.

Planning domestic arrangements for the meeting

This is best carried out by the secretary and includes:

*   The venue: This should be comfortable, convenient for members and as far as possible free from interruptions and noise.
*   A secretary to take notes during the meeting: The chairperson should never attempt to take notes as this will cause the meeting to break down. Asking a member to be the note-taker is also contraindicated, as this could lead to a conflict of interests arising.
*   Organizing visual aids for short presentations during the meeting:. These include overhead projector, flipboard, slide projector or video recorder and television. Selected visual aids should be planned well in advance to ensure their availability, and must be checked prior to the meeting to ensure they are in proper working order.

Pre meeting briefing

Immediately prior to the meeting it is a good idea for the chairperson and secretary to get together for a short briefing session. Fifteen minutes is usually sufficient to outline how the meeting will progress and to go through papers, reports etc. for distribution.

Opening the meeting

The chairperson should be ready to welcome members in a warm and friendly manner and to open the meeting. This will help to create the right atmosphere, inspire confidence and command respect. The introductory statement summarizing the purpose of the meeting is given. Apologies of members who are unable to attend are recorded. When there are notes or minutes of a previous meeting these are checked for accuracy and agreed as a true record.

Conducting the meeting

The chairperson should not do all the talking, but must ensure everyone has the opportunity to participate At the same time certain members must not be allowed to dominate. There are a number of techniques that are helpful for controlling a meeting which include:

- when a person is too talkative the chairperson can interrupt with something like 'that's an interesting point ... what do other members think about this ?' or 'that's interesting...perhaps we could discuss this further outside the meeting'.
- when emotions get high the chairperson must keep control by emphasizing points of agreement and minimizing points of disagreement. Another technique is to remind members of the purpose of the meeting and bring the meeting back into focus again.
- when discussion goes off the subject this could indicate a lack of interest. The chairperson can summarize what has already been said to help keep the discussion on course.
- if the chairperson suspects there may be a personality clash during the meeting it may be advisable to talk to certain members beforehand. They can be politely asked to 'leave any negative feelings they have to each other outside the meeting'.
- when a member appears timid and shy and has not contributed the chairperson can encourage their involvement by asking a question which they will be able to answer.
- when members engage in side-conversation or whisper amongst themselves the chairperson can direct a question to one of them, and restate the last comment made to the meeting. A reminder that only one meeting can be held at a time would not be amiss.
- when a member has difficulty in expressing what they mean the chairperson can either rephrase what that person has said and then ask for confirmation, or help that person to say what they mean without being patronizing.

It is important the chairperson summarizes at the end of each agenda item for the benefit of members and to help the notetaker.

Concluding the meeting

The chairperson ends the meeting when all the agenda items have been discussed, explored and summarized, and each member has been asked if they have any other business or questions.

Notes of the meeting

It is essential that some form of record is produced:
- detailed minutes are usually required for formal committee meetings.
- notes are usually more suitable for the majority of meetings.
- notes or minutes must be accurate and not a verbatim report, and produced quickly - if possible within five working days.
- the notes (or minutes) will be structured according to the agenda.
- there should be an 'action column' to identify which members or groups are required to carry out certain action as a result of decisions made during the meeting.
- the secretary should produce a 'draft copy' within three days after the meeting ready for the chairperson to scan and approve.
- the notes (or minutes) are distributed and circulated to those who attended the meeting or who sent apologies. Also to wards, departments and clinical areas, and senior managers and directors as appropriate.

Summary

Communication is the most important skill in management. Effective communication is the key to success in any organization. For midwifery managers the challenge of effective communication is two-fold. Firstly to use sound communication processes themselves, and secondly to facilitate others to communicate effectively with mothers and their families, colleagues and other health professionals.

Communication is a two way process which involves a sender and a receiver. There are five steps in the communication process. Frequently things go wrong , barriers are created and communication breaks down.

Fundamentally communications can be classified into verbal, written and non verbal. Verbal communication can be face to face or by telephone. Effective verbal communication requires proper preparation, clarity of speech and the ability to tune into the 'world of the listener'. The listener is required to listen actively, but most people are unable to give close attention for more than sixty seconds. Skills in the art of listening must be learned and developed. The way a person responds to another will affect communication. When positive the person is encouraged, when negative communication can break down.

Non verbal communication is the language of the body. It is intentional or unintentional when clues are given about how a person feels without their knowing. Interpreting non verbal signals is essential for effective communication because they reveal much about a person, and can intensify or reduce interaction.

The written word is a permanent record. Writing is a good medium for messages: letters, memos, records, reports and notices. It can be conveyed on paper or by electronic systems. Careful planning is necessary to assess the purpose of writing, who will read it, what to write and how to present it. Once written, there is little opportunity to clarification and explanation, and it is open to ambiguity. Writing reports are an essential part of the managerial process because findings and proposals have a strong impact on decision making.

As midwifery managers take on more responsibility in the flattened management structure they will find themselves more frequently chairing and conducting meetings. The role of the chairperson is critical to the success of the meeting. Meetings must be carefully planned and conducted in a way to encourage participation of all the members. Records of meetings must be accurate, include an 'action column' and be distributed promptly.

CHAPTER EIGHT

The Cost of Quality

'Quality isn't a process - it's a state of mind'.
(David Young, Managing Director, Kineticon.)

Today, in the National Health Service, quality and 'value for money' are the overriding factors that will secure future contracts for NHS Trusts. Needless to say quality is at the top of each Trust's agenda. Moreover, quality has been at the top of the political agenda throughout the last decade.

The changes that came about as a result of *Working for Patients* (1989) have endorsed this preoccupation with quality, and at the same time reformed the way care is provided in the National Health Service. The main reason given for implementing *Working for Patients* was to provide a service that puts patients first. What these changes have actually shown is a move to make the National Health Service more businesslike by putting the consumer first - the business approach being based on successes in the industrial and commercial sector. In theory, benefits for health service users cannot be disputed if receiving high quality health care is the objective. In practice, measures are unsophisticated and therefore effectiveness is difficult to examine.

Health care professionals will say standards and quality have always been important. They maintain they act in the best interest of patients within the resources available to them, but as Jacquerye (1994) observes 'only a few will challenge the objectivity of this'. Further she argues that health care managers are confronted with similar problems, and says it is their responsibility to see their institutions provide adequate personnel and resources to ensure a specific level of care can be delivered.

Midwifery managers and midwives have generally given their support to the concept of providing a high quality service for all mothers and babies. Also mothers and their families expect high standards in modern times. Fundamentally, this is the message conveyed in the booklet *NHS The Patient Charter Maternity Services* (1995), part of the Citizens Charter campaign to raise standards. Quality is also at the heart *Changing Childbirth* (1993) reforms, making maternity care more consumer responsive and making women equal partners in their care.

Demands for improved quality in health care will continue unabated, not only from the consumers of health care and their representatives, but from health professionals, managers and politicians. Quality is now the language of the National Health Service.

Quality is the buzz word for success but what exactly does quality mean? Is there a universal meaning, or does quality mean different things to different people?

The meaning of quality

According to Munro-Faure (1992) quality is one of the most misunderstood issues in business today, and yet it is central to the survival of even the largest organization. Defining quality is difficult because people perceive quality in different ways. Like most issues in life the views on quality are diverse. At one end of the spectrum is the thought that quality is too ill defined to be able to measure and quantify. That to actually attempt to measure it would be to impair it, and to formally plan its improvement would be to completely destroy it.. Whereas Handy (Fardell, 1994) says 'quality like truth is an attitude of mind. It does not come easily. It needs the right equipment, the right people and the right environment'.

As to the meaning of quality opinions are widespread and can range from representing:

- richness, luxury, beauty
- value for money
- freedom from pain and discomfort
- living a long life
- goodness, respect, kindness.

Most people, however, still seem to equate quality with expense. Slogans such a 'providing a Rolls Royce service' have been used to promote this, but this does not explain why a person who can afford to buy a Rolls Royce will buy a Ford car instead? Both are described as quality products, so the key must be in the satisfaction level provided by fulfilling what the customer needed. Putting it simply, as Auld (1992) asserts 'quality is about meeting customer requirements'. Yet is it possible this elementary message is deceptively too simple?

Who are the customers of the National Health Service? Are customers the same as users? When we apply the complex issue of customers to Maternity Services, we find there are three types:

- customers who are recipients of care - the mothers and babies, clients
- customers who are users of maternity services
  - external (mothers and babies)
  - internal (midwives, obstetricians, neonatologists, paediatricians and other health workers
- customers who purchase maternity services on behalf of clients
  - the Health Authorities
  - general practitioners

For clarity it is simpler to divide customers of Maternity Services into two:

- external - mothers and babies and purchasers of maternity services
- internal - midwifery, medical and support services staff

Can quality be defined?

The Oxford English Dictionary defines quality as 'a degree of excellence' and the Chambers 20th Century Dictionary as a 'high grade of excellence'. The agreement of the word 'excellence' has become related to effectiveness and closeness to the customer. Hence the use of 'excellence' in many of the slogans during the 1980s. The British Standards Institute (Morgan, 1994) recommended that any usage of the term should involve:

> 'a degree of excellence; reflect on measurement of a product in terms of departure from an ideal and demonstrate fitness for purpose relating to the ability to meet stated needs'.

However, Kanter and Mirvis (Howe, Gaeddert and Howe, 1993) claimed that rhetoric about excellence was well ahead of reality in most organizations.

Koch (1993) admits quality is difficult to define, but by no means impossible. He believes that the model, partly developed by Maxwell in 1984 explains adequately the six dimensions of quality. These are particularly pertinent to the National Health Service which is designed to meet customer needs and expectations (Fig. 8.1).

- acceptability
- equity
- appropriateness
- efficiency
- effectiveness
- accessibility

Fig. 8.1: Six dimensions of quality for health care

Equally these dimensions can be applied in turn. At every stage of care for all users of the National Health Service as follows:

- the actual care provided - within a speciality(ies) and the service as a whole
- what information is offered and given and how it is elicited
- the way information is communicated
- the attitude of health professionals and support workers, whilst providing care and during communication
- the physical environment of the hospital or health service premises - where care and information is given and received.

Maternity Service measures of success will be dependent on maternity outcomes, the provision of effective care for each mother and baby, and from consumer feedback. The responsibility for ensuring continued quality and improvements in each of the above dimensions will rest with all maternity staff - midwifery managers, professionals and support workers at every level. Clearly, the first aim is to provide high quality maternity care to the customers - the mothers and babies, and satisfy the purchasers. The second aim is to ensure that the internal customers, work in an open culture, have the right skills and the right equipment and are able to provide high quality care.

Total Quality Management (TQM)

Total Quality Management has fast become the business philosophy of the 1990s. It links the provider and customer through satisfying the customer's requirements as efficiently and profitably as possible. It embraces every activity carried out by every employee in the organization.

The concept of TQM includes:

- a corporate management approach which recognizes that customer needs and business goals are inseparable.

- a commitment which originates at Chief Executive and top management level and is promoted throughout the organization and is integral to all activities.

- putting into place arrangements and systems which will:
  - cultivate quality
  - reduce duplication
  - prevent errors
  - ensure every aspect of the service is aligned to the needs of its customers external and internal.

- involving every aspect of the service and the active dedication of all the staff to meet the customers needs.

- agreeing and setting standards and regularly carrying out clinical and service audits.

- monitoring customer satisfaction; understanding customer needs and monitoring changing expectations - through regular reviews and audits.

- providing resources to develop quality and act as role models; and processes that are capable of delivering and measuring the specified service consistently through flexible procedures and information systems.

The quality chain

It can be seen that TQM ensures maximum effectiveness and efficiency within an organization, but this can only be achieved if every part works together as a complete entity. The interdependence of every person actively affecting each other is at the core of the internal customer concept and the customer-supplier chain. The quality chain is based on the fact that every organization consists of a chain of suppliers and customers. Everyone in this system is at once a customer and supplier of the person before and after in the chain. If at any time a link is weak or breaks down, for example a member of staff or piece of equipment does not meet the standards, failures will become apparent (Fig. 8.2).

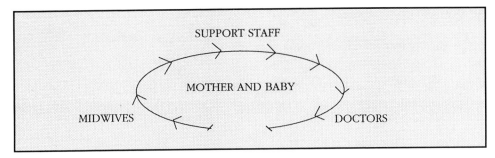

Fig. 8.2: Showing just one break in the chain could result in failure to meet the customers needs

For TQM to be effective the following functions have to be met:

* understanding customers
* understanding each specialist service function
* continuous quality improvement
* use of quality tools.

A breakdown of each of these functions is shown in Figure 8.3.

TOTAL QUALITY MANAGEMENT			
Understanding customers **- External** **- Internal**	**Understanding Maternity Services function**	**Continuous improvement**	**Quality tools**
Know your customers	involves: • function analysis • quality costs when needs are not met the first time costs can be high: • complaints • litigation	requires: • commitment by managers • involving staff • in service education • continuing education • teamworking • preventing errors • evaluation • audit • consumer surveys and feedback	include: • statistics • eliminating problems • skilled practitioners • quality awards • success stories • media publications

Fig. 8.3 Showing total quality 'in action'

TQM in summary requires:

- quality leadership
- total commitment
- active involvement of everyone in the organization.

It involves creating a participative environment for staff and developing a team approach to:

- create a quality policy that is linked to the business plan
- motivate and promote ownership
- break down professional barriers
- share knowledge, skills and expertise.

Commitment and vision by themselves are not enough. Uncoordinated action plans can lead to chaos. The vital key is recognizing and understanding the supplier-customer interface, and managing the organization in such a way that customer needs are met, both external and internal.

The main benefits of introducing TQM are:

- it provides services that meet customer needs
- it reduces complaints through providing staff with the right skills and attitudes, and eliminating errors
- it raises the image of the NHS Trust and the Maternity Services
- external customers will want to use the Maternity Services
- it improves staff morale through improved job satisfaction because they work in a NHS Trust and Maternity Services with a good reputation
- purchasers will be committed to renew contracts, and there will be increased opportunities to secure additional contracts with new purchasers.

Implementing Total Quality Management in the NHS

According to Morgan (1994) there are varying opinions as to the progress of implementing TQM in the public service. He says it has been argued that most are now in the 'Awakening Stage' as described by Crosby (Morgan, 1994). This indicates that managers in the National Health Service are just beginning to recognize that quality management is useful. They are prepared to invest only a limited amount of time and money, and tend to resolve problems on an ad hoc basis. Morgan believes much more will have to be done by NHS Trusts if they are committed to providing a health service that meets customers needs.

Education and training

The only way to successfully implement a clear quality policy is through education and in-service training. TQM starts with and continues through education and training. Only then will everyone begin to understand the concepts and processes that form the basis of quality improvement. No one should be excluded, whatever their position and where they fit in the organization. Everyone needs to know and understand how they can work together in the quality chain for providing a service which meets the needs of both external and internal customers.

Part of the training will be to identify the right Total Quality Programme to fit the business and service goals of the NHS Trust and its culture. This is done by creating and sharing a vision which is accepted and owned by the staff, and by agreeing what skills are required to provide the service at all levels.

Other elements of training will include:

1.   Promoting a climate which is supportive of critical evaluation, innovation and change.

2.   Teambuilding and teamworking. It is only through effective teamwork that problems will be identified, solved and prevented. TQM seeks to create a culture in which everyone is continuously evaluating and improving their work.

3.   Learning about the stages of TQM:
     - planning for quality
     - involving external and internal customers
     - marketing
     - inspection: screening and checking processes
     - quality control:
            techniques and activities for monitoring performance
            setting standards
            systems that find and eliminate problems
            clinical and medical audit
     - quality improvement
            consumer suggestions
            consumer feedback and surveys
            research
            clinical risk management and reporting systems
            working with patient associations and representatives
            increasing resources
            contracts with purchasers

Quality and the midwife manager

The midwifery manager is the key person to facilitate the creation of a quality culture in Maternity Services. Of course this must 'dovetail' with the NHS Trust's corporate culture and merge with the Total Quality Management programme. In addition both the *Changing Childbirth* (1993) recommendations and guidance in the NHS Patients Charter booklet *Maternity Services* (1995), have given more scope for developing a high quality service, which is sensitive to meeting the needs of mothers and babies.

Ways and mechanisms for midwifery managers to achieve quality Maternity Services include:

- promoting a climate that is conducive to change
- motivating staff and getting them committed to meeting consumer needs
- reading as much as you can about quality - articles, books, research etc.
- circulating information and articles on quality
- making quality a regular agenda item along with business goals and plans
- asking and encouraging staff to initiate ideas for quality improvement
- being receptive to new ideas and not throwing them out because they were not your idea
- involving midwives - and yourself - in self assessment, clinical audit, consumer satisfaction surveys and consumer suggestions and feedback
- involving midwives - and yourself - in local and national quality initiatives and research
- promoting and supporting 'Quality Circles'
- knowing when it is right to consult others before making a decision
- providing continuing and in-service education on 'Quality' and 'Communication' through study days, workshops, discussions etc.
- encouraging staff to attend external study days, and visit other Maternity and neonatal Services to bring back new ideas for sharing with colleagues, users and yourself.

Some of the most important issues involving quality are the ones to which Handy alludes to when he says:

> 'Quality like truth is an attitude of mind. It does not come easily. It needs the right equipment, the right people and the right environment'.

Is quality an attitude of mind? Do midwives perceive quality as something separate and additional to what they already do? Some midwives have been heard to say they haven't time for quality, but what do they mean? Until the concept of quality is accepted that it means the same as meeting consumer needs and expectations, then midwives will continue to have trouble with the quality issue. Quality is an attitude of mind. Midwives who work in a Maternity Service culture that is open and caring will be encouraged to demonstrate positive attitudes, and will live and breathe quality in everything they do.

Who are the right people? Midwives are central to the provision of maternity care, and are continuously involved in the care of mothers and babies, throughout a twenty four hour cycle. Because of this they are best placed for ensuring the crucial quality aspect of care is achieved. Today, mothers and their families expect competent compassionate care from midwives, and most midwives respond by providing this. The 'Named Midwife' arrangement is an excellent way for enhancing the quality of care. Yet this alone is not sufficient. Research is showing that proficient midwifery practice benefits maternal and neonatal care the most. Skilled midwifery care is not a luxury, but essential for providing quality by meeting the needs of mothers and babies.

Whose responsibility is it for providing the right equipment and the right environment? The midwifery manager, working collaboratively with midwives must assess that they have the proper resources, the right skills and the appropriate procedures in place to do their jobs well (see Management of Resources - Chapter 5). Also by creating a more 'homelike' environment in the Maternity Unit, mothers and their families will be helped to feel more relaxed.

Ways to involve staff in continuous evaluation and improvement

Generally there two types of teams that are useful for facilitating problem solving associated with quality. These are:

- Temporary: teams that are created to deal with specific problems. These can be external (a team which is 'bought in') or internal ('a quality circle').

- Permanent: teams that are part of the workforce who meet for brainstorming or Pareto analysis.

Brain storming

This is a good method for getting staff to generate and produce ideas. It can also be used for identifying the possible causes of a problem, as well as considering ways of how the problem can be solved. Brain storming has two stages:

1. The first stage involves getting people to share their ideas, and listing each one. The use of a flipboard greatly facilitates brain storming because the more ideas people can see displayed the more enthusiastic they become to provide even more ideas. The aim is to get as many ideas as possible. These are recorded in no specific order and without evaluation.

2. The second stage entails the group evaluating each idea in turn and assessing how feasible they are. These are then prioritized with possible courses of action.

Pareto analysis

This can be used for evaluating a list of possible reasons as to why quality is not being achieved. The analysis is based on a principle produced by the 19th century Italian economist and sociologist Vilfredo Pareto, who stated that only a small number of items, tasks or behaviours in a group are significant. Juran (Morgan, 1994) called these the 'vital few' and the remainder of the items he called the 'trivial many'.

Pareto analysis is, therefore, an attempt to separate the trivial problems from the vital few. Trivial problems are estimated to take up 80 per cent of a group's time but produce only 20 per cent positive results. The vital few problems take up only 20 per cent of the group's time but produce 80 per cent of the positive results. By identifying the vital few greater progress can be made in improving the quality of the service.

Quality circles

'A quality circle is a small group of people from the same work area that voluntarily meets on a regular basis to identify, analyze, and solve problems of various types'. (Quality Circle Digest, Red Bluff, USA).

Quality circles were developed in Japan in 1961 by Dr K Ishikawa and the Union of Japanese Scientists and Engineers (JUSE) by combining behavioural sciences together with quality sciences. The latter had been introduced as a result of a collapsed post-war Japan. The phenomenon of quality circles grew in Japan to involve millions of employees. During the 1970s quality circles spread to the western world where quality, alongside price and delivery formed the basis on which companies established themselves and maintained their markets.

In the United Kingdom, as a result of the *Griffiths Report* (1983), changes in accountability and resource restrictions forced National Health Service managers to review their management style. Consequently, quality circles have been tried with varying levels of success.

CHARACTERISTICS OF A QUALITY CIRCLE
Ideally members should be from the same work area, perform similar work or interact closely to get a job done. In this way problems they select will be familiar to them all.

Membership is strictly voluntary. No one is required to participate and no one is kept out. Membership can range from 'three to thirteen members' (Song, 1981).

A quality circle is made up of four interrelated parts:

• the members themselves
• the circle leader
• the facilitator (programme co-ordinator)
• the NHS Trust Quality Team

There is no limit to the number of circles that can take place in a given area. As many circles as are needed can be formed and to accommodate all who want to join.

Most circles meet for one hour each week, but the time can vary accordingly. Sometimes they can be as short as thirty minutes.

A circle will work through a sequence of stages:

• identification of a number of problems
• selection - by the group - of the problem with the highest priority
• collection of data required
• analysis of the problem
• possible solutions
• selection of recommendations for solving the problem
• presentation of findings and recommendations to the manager or managers.

Circles are urged to concern themselves with quality issues only. Problems that directly affect working conditions may be acceptable if not already the concern of the joint consultative committee or unions.

Each circle has its own code of conduct, and meetings will be conducted in a businesslike manner.

Each participant in the circle will receive training as follows:

- The facilitator - usually the midwifery manager or midwifery sister - will be trained in the theory and practice of quality circles, and will act as a support to the circle. She will ensure members can meet in work time or get the time made up, have the use of a suitable room for meetings and where to obtain data for the problem analysis. The facilitator will greatly influence the success of the circle.
- The circle leader - will be trained by the facilitator in group dynamics and how to chair meetings
- The circle members - will be trained by the circle leader in brainstorming, cause and effect and analytical problem-solving.

The facilitator attends, or is available for, most circle meetings and is the link between circles, the Maternity Services and senior management.

The concept of Quality Circles usually gains quicker acceptance when it fits into the existing structure and culture. Management support is essential. According to Song (1981) unless 'top management believes a quality circle programme will benefit the organization and support it, the programme will not be effective'.

In the circle's presentation to the midwifery manager and other managers, each member will participate in presenting their analysis, findings and recommendations with the use of charts, diagrams etc. The presentation usually serves as a powerful stimulus to the circle members as well as the managers. However, the decision to implement rests with management. When proposals are accepted circle members should play an active part in implementation.

The benefits of quality circles are that they:

- improve the services to customers
- inspire more effective teamwork
- increase staff motivation
- promote job and work involvement
- improve communications
- create problem-solving capability
- create a perspective of problem-prevention
- promote leadership development
- harmonize manager and staff relations.

What everyone can do to achieve quality

- think constantly about quality
- plan carefully and pay attention to detail in everything you do
- know as much as you can:
  - before providing actual care to each mother and baby
  - when communicating with mothers and their relatives, colleagues and visitors
  - when doing a job, a procedure or task
- have the right attitude towards meeting the needs of customers
- set and agree standards, own them and prevent problems
- evaluate everything you do and learn from difficulties and mistakes
- make your goal 100 per cent for quality
- develop the 'team spirit' and share ideas and successes with others
- be proud and enjoy what you do
- take initiatives and accept new challenges
- have a sense of humour.

Does quality pay?

For quality to make a lasting impact, every section of the NHS Trust has to be focused on customer commitment and not just satisfaction.

Lessons about quality can be learned from the USA. Throughout the 1980s quality programmes were implemented in America and there are some parallels in the way quality has been introduced in the National Health Service.

According to Howe et al. (1993) research carried out on quality programmes in America's top thousand corporations, suggested that most companies were forced to join the 'quality revolution' due to a crisis within their industry or company. The significance of this was they had a 'crisis quality mentality', which pushed the organization in many directions at the same time. On a macro level it appeared quality was paying, but appearances can be deceptive. On closer inspection many of the quality initiatives remained 'parallel activities' that never became fully integrated into the everyday business of the company. The concept and value of customer commitment was not integrated into the ongoing business practices.

Only when 'quality and business objectives are invisibly linked' will quality pay.

The following salutary tale supports this link. It is a true account edited from *Quality on Trial* (1993), which sums up the integration of quality and business. It is given to demonstrate what true integration of quality and business really means, and will be of value to midwifery managers and midwives in planning quality Maternity Services.

'The vice-president of quality assurance for an industrial organization was showing his last slide. Proudly he said "This is the culmination of our second year of quality". The slide showed the company had fifty quality teams meeting regularly, ten quality awards had been made to employees who submitted the best quality suggestions, and all employees had been trained in TQM.

He went on to say "Most of our plants are well along the way to establishing quality processes - with one notable exception". He turned to the general manager of this plant - the most successful section in the division - and asked "why is your group the only one that isn't meeting its quality process objectives?"

"Well" the manager replied slowly "we really don't talk all that much about quality processes".

Every head in the room jerked up.

"Let me understand you" said the vice-president in carefully measured tones, "every other plant is meeting its objectives of implementing quality processes - and you're telling me your section isn't doing anything".

"That's not what I said" - the manager seemed surprisingly unruffled - "What I said was we don't talk that much about quality processes. We're usually talking about our business objectives. For us, quality and business objectives are invisibly linked".

'Vision for the Future'

In the climate of quality, purchasing and providing, it was befitting that the document *Vision for the Future* (1993) was published. In the preface, Yvonne Moores, Chief Nursing Officer and Director of Nursing of the NHS Management Executive, states the document provides a vision for the nursing, midwifery and health visiting contribution to health and health care. The document gives a considered view of the future of the National Health Service, and identifies five key areas and twelve targets which are designed to help practitioners provide high quality health care and to improve the health of the population.

The first of these key areas is quality, outcomes and audit. This clearly focuses on the requirement to meet the needs of patients, and to fulfil the rights, and national and local standards within the *Patients' Charter* (1993). Nursing and midwifery professionals are reminded that delivery of high quality cost effective care is central to the philosophy of their professions, and that they must ensure their work, where possible, is research based good practice. Continuous evaluation is essential to good practice, and standards must be amended in response to evaluations into the process and outcome of care.

The quality targets are summarized as follows:

- Individualized patient care: systems of care must demonstrate that a named nurse, midwife or health visitor is personally identified as having responsibility for care and its delivery, engaging other practitioners as needs demand.

- Shared protocols and shared care planning: with consumers, professional colleagues and managers. Clients should be involved as fully as possible in the planning and delivery of care.

- Uni- and multi-disciplinary clinical audit: nurses, midwives and health visitors should participate in clinical audit and standards of practice must be adjusted in response to such evaluations.

- High quality cost-effective care: should take account of resource management and value for money initiatives, and ensure that the professionals and the infrastructure are able to deliver the most effective 'skill-mix'.

- Research based practice: every nurse, midwife and health visitor should be able to recognize the role of research and research based knowledge in the delivery of high quality care.

- Purchasing of health care: purchasing organizations should review their arrangements for ensuring high quality informed professional advice, and recognize the contribution that appropriately skilled nurses, midwives and health visitors can make to the purchasing cycle.

- Professional education and training: planning should remain an important part of the management agenda, and health care providers and educational institutions must ensure that pre and post registration programmes meet changing service needs.

How midwives can encourage a quality health service

- Midwives must recognize they are in a prime position to encourage and nurture quality, and this can be done by working closely with their midwifery managers, the NHS Trust Director of Nursing and Midwifery and with each other.

- They must attempt to organize and encourage debate about health care. This will allow them to be involved in the development of strategies for Maternity Services that do not separate the purchaser and provider.

- Midwives must accept that 'decision-making in health care can be a difficult, and sometimes painful, process' (Deighan , 1993). It involves resolving cost and organizational problems, while frequently 'care issues' remain with the professionals.

- Midwives must understand that effective management - both managing the Maternity Services and providing direct care to mothers and babies - entails the identification and measurement of clinical outcomes within contracts. This is fundamental to quality improvement.

- Midwives must accept that quality is the issue that will unite them with other professionals. Quality is a great equaliser - it does allow for professional rivalry but concentrates on the needs of the consumers.

- Midwives must continue to take lead positions in health care planning, monitoring and education, and move into positions of service and business planning, contracting and marketing. This will ensure quality will 'market' the Maternity Services, and not only financial issues.

- Midwives must read, understand and work towards quality and the targets in the *Vision for the Future* (1993). They must ensure managers and other professional groups listen to them, and act on what they say.

Obtaining information from customers

The process of acquiring information from maternity services customers is central to 'customer relations'. This is not just because it is a principal way of finding out whether the needs of customers are being met, but because it shows customers are valued and important. Obtaining information involves collecting customers views and acting upon the findings. Being seen to act is the most important aspect of obtaining consumer feedback.

For customers to have confidence in their local health services, NHS Trusts must show they are meeting users needs. Lack of confidence of users and purchasers and other negative emotions, will seriously damage relations between health service staff and their customers.

Involving customers in the planning of maternity services

There are many ways to obtain customer information, and these include:

- surveys
- questionnaires
- structured interviews
- voluntary feedback.

Usually these methods tend to concentrate on obtaining information from individual mothers who have used, or are currently using the Maternity Services.

For planning future changes in Maternity Services, it is important to obtain the opinions of individual mothers and staff and also the views of different sections of the community. Emphasis is now on 'building in the customer voice' when planning and reviewing services. Consumer ideas can be obtained by involving representatives who speak for others, using market research techniques, through postal research and by arranging local health forums.

The opinions of groups such as the Community Health Council (CHC), and voluntary organizations associated with maternity and neonatal care, are invaluable for planning and critically reviewing local Maternity Services. However, difficulties can sometimes arise with consumer representatives. Members of voluntary bodies represent the needs and wishes of a certain category of customer. Also there is a tendency to only represent the views of those with a particular interest or perspective of the services. According to McIver and Carr-Hill (1989), representatives 'speaking from the point of view of their particular customers, will be partisan where planning is concerned'. Another difficulty with representatives, is the type of person most likely to join a voluntary organization or committee. They are generally white, of mature age and middle class. The danger is that certain voluntary groups, those with the most effective and strong representation, will gain over the weaker groups and those not represented, such as ethnic minorities and teenagers. To overcome these problems it is necessary to ensure the views of all categories of people are obtained. This includes present customers and potential customers. This does not devalue the views of the local voluntary groups, such as the National Childbirth Trust (NCT), Stillbirth and Neonatal Death Society (SANDS). On the contrary, by involving other sections of the community this will give a more balanced outlook in the planning of Maternity Services.

How to set up and conduct a consumer survey

Undertaking a consumer survey is a complex process. Before embarking on the survey decisions have to be made about how long it will take, what resources are needed, how much it will cost, and the possible pitfalls - so these can be avoided. Careful design and preliminary checks are necessary to ensure the survey is successful.

The following step by step guide outlines the main activities involved in carrying out a survey:

REASON FOR SURVEY

Decide on the purpose of the survey, specify the precise aims and objectives and what information is required. These are the essential preliminary elements. The type of study used for obtaining consumer feedback is usually known as a 'descriptive study'. Although descriptive, it still has to have well defined objectives. Information and consumer feedback is only useful when the objectives for the survey are clear.

PROMOTING INTEREST AND GAINING SUPPORT

Talk to as many people as possible about the proposed survey. Explain the reasons for the study - for example 'to obtain the views of mothers about their care during the postnatal period, to decide whether changes are required in the way postnatal care is provided and to decide priorities for action'. Consult with midwifery, medical and senior colleagues and elicit their help. Identify which aspects the survey will focus on. Estimate the amount of interest, and particularly the effect the survey will have on the service. Even the most conclusive survey is wasted if it is unread, the proposals are rejected, or the report sits on a shelf and is forgotten.

DESIGN PREPARATION

Decide on the design of the survey. Check to see if similar surveys have been carried out, and write and obtain information. From these and your own questions, compile a questionnaire. A recommended format by the University of York (1989) is an average of five pre-coded questions per section, and five sections for each area to be surveyed.

For example, the survey on 'postnatal care' will focus on three areas. These can be divided as follows:

1.   education and guidance given to mothers in caring for their new baby
2.   support and help given to mothers whilst feeding their baby
3.   the amount of choice each mother had regarding her transfer home from hospital.

This would amount to a fifteen section questionnaire.

Allow for open comments in some of the sections. Although the questionnaire may appear long, the advantage is that it enables research in the three main areas to be covered in considerable detail. Also more general opinions can be collected about the postnatal services.

PILOTING

Get the draft questionnaire typed and test a small sample of mothers in two different environments. For example, a small group of mothers just prior to leaving the postnatal ward, and a small number in their own homes who have had community midwifery care. Some mothers will find the questionnaire satisfactory whilst others will find it complicated. Also seek the views of midwifery and medical colleagues.

Produce a second version of the questionnaire and test again in one area. With minor modifications this will become the final version. Also include an introductory paragraph explaining why the survey is being carried out and how to return the questionnaire.

PRACTICAL ARRANGEMENTS

Prepare sufficient numbers of questionnaires for distribution. Remind midwives of the survey and ask for their help by being available should mothers encounter any difficulties. This is especially relevant if the pilot study identified that some mothers experienced difficulties.

Distribute questionnaires with the help of the staff, or involving voluntary helpers, such as the local National Childbirth Trust. Each mother is invited to participate and a questionnaire is handed to the mother individually, with a personal explanation about the survey. A record should be kept of mothers who refuse to participate so the non-response rate can be calculated. Envelopes are provided to ensure confidentiality. Arrange for collection, in boxes prominently situated in the wards, or via a postal arrangement addressed to the survey organizer. This is necessary for mothers in their own home. Completed questionnaires are collected from boxes every three days. All uncompleted questionnaires should be collected and counted.

DATA CODING AND ENTRY

Draw up a coding scheme for 'associated open comments' and add to the pre-coded questions. Decide how to summarize other open comments, or to report on them verbatim. With the use a computerized system, data can be entered, coded and analysed. Without the use of a computer it is possible to code, analyse and report manually. This may be time consuming but usually the advantages of conducting the survey, reporting and acting on its findings will far outweigh the time and effort.

REPORTING

Provide a two-page summary of the main results, which includes the distinct views of different groups of mothers. Present remarks on the replies of the more focused questions and the open comments. Observations should be noted and recommendations made. A report of around twenty pages, including the summary, is sufficient to gain people's interest and get the survey-report noticed and talked about.

Send thank you letters to staff involved in the survey. The final report should be discussed and shared with staff. A copy of the report should be circulated widely, to senior managers and consumer representatives, and a copy held in each ward, department and sections of the community.

PRESENTATION OF FINDINGS

Give several presentations on the findings of the study. Set up a small working group to consider the outcome of the survey, its recommendations and how to implement agreed changes for improving the services. When ready to release news of the proposed changes involve the local media (newspapers, radio and television).

Summary

Providing quality services and 'value for money' are the overriding factors that will secure future contracts for NHS Trusts.

Defining quality is difficult and diverse opinions exist. Nevertheless quality is central to the success of all organizations. Fundamentally quality is about meeting customer requirements, but the customer concept is complex in the NHS. External customers are both users of health care- the patients and clients, and the purchasers, - the health authorities and GP Fundholders, who acquire contracts and purchase on behalf of the users. Internal customers are the professional, managerial and support staff who provide services.

Maxwell's six dimensions of quality are pertinent to the provision of NHS care and provide a system for assessing standards, communications and the physical environment of hospitals and health buildings.

Total Quality Management (TQM) is the business philosophy of the 1990s. It links the providers of health care and customers through satisfying the customers requirements as efficiently and profitably as possible. TQM is a corporate approach and involves every member of staff and every activity in the NHS Trust. It recognizes that customer needs and business goals are inseparable.

Teamworking is essential for continuous evaluation and raising of standards. Quality Circles provide a forum for small teams to solve work related problems, recommend solutions and implement improvements. Individuals can achieve quality in their daily work by having the right attitude and developing personal techniques to monitor their standards.

Delivery of 'high quality cost effective care is central to the philosophy of the nursing midwifery and health visitors' (*Vision for the Future*, 1993). Midwives can encourage a quality service by recognizing that their practice needs to be competent and research based. Skilled midwifery care is not a luxury but essential for providing a quality service which meets the needs of mothers and babies.

Obtaining information from customers is a way of assessing whether their health needs have been met. Also it shows their views are valued. Involving potential customers and sections of the community when planning and reviewing health services will provide ideas and expectations, which can be used in conjunction with those of health workers. Conducting a consumer survey may be an elaborate process, but with careful preparation, systemic data collection and succinct report writing, recommendations can be implemented and benefits realized.

CHAPTER NINE

Ethics

'Understanding another person is more than feeling sympathy and empathy. To understand others we need to understand how we operate as meaning-creating creatures, how we each experience ourselves and our world'. (Dorothy Rowe, 1992)

Does ethics concern midwifery managers?

During the last two decades there has been increased concern with the ethical management of organizations in society, ranging from central government to the NHS Trusts responsible for providing health care at local level.

For the midwifery manager a special type of moral leadership is called upon, which includes responsibility for:

- social and ethical decision-making
- contributing to formulation of policies and practices
- assisting with resource allocation and monitoring resources
- involving fairness and concern for others
- supporting and leading others through ethical dilemmas.

Modern midwifery practice abounds with value-laden situations where conflicts can arise, and this requires managerial leadership to enable sound ethical decisions to be made. Although ethical dilemmas in midwifery practice do not occur regularly, they need to be recognized and carefully defined, so that the way they are dealt with can be discussed and debated on known principles of ethics.

Whistle-blowing is slowly becoming accepted in the National Health Service. The document 'Guidance for Staff on Relations with the Public and Media' (1993) issued by the NHS Management Executive Board, promised whistle-blowing would be made easier, but a survey carried out in November 1994 showed many health workers would be unlikely to speak out about misconduct or malpractice.

Although midwifery managers operate at the centre of a clinical work environment which is influenced by different attitudes and assumptions, and where judgements are made, they must not lose sight of their management responsibilities. Maternity Services goals have to be met, and sometimes in the drive to achieve these, the midwifery manager will come into conflict with midwives, medical colleagues and mothers. The dilemma for midwifery managers is that they have responsibilities to many groups of people at one time, and it is difficult to please them all. These include:

- mothers and babies
- midwifery and support service staff
- the Clinical Director
- medical colleagues; professions allied to maternity care
- senior NHS Trust managers.

According to Wall (1989) ethics are 'not just a framework of protective rules,' nor are they necessarily the same as the law. Neither are they remote or abstract. On the contrary, managers face the challenge of doing what is right every day in their hospitals, organizations and offices.

Defining ethics and morality

Philosophers through the ages have defined ethics as a set of standards, or principles of conduct, which govern the behaviour of an individual, or a group of individuals.

Ethics are generally concerned with questions of right and wrong, or with moral duties (Maloney, 1994). The term ethics is always used in the plural. As Hosmer (Maloney, 1994) points out this is because people have a 'system of beliefs' by which they live, and not just one single value.

Morality, according to Hosmer, is a set of standards by which people judge one another. Viewed another way, morals are the way people expect others to behave, according to established group norms. A further dimension has been added to morality by Aroskar (Maloney, 1994) which is moral conduct, 'not what is actually done but what ought to be done'. She looked into the constraints which act as barriers in the roles of nurse managers, and cited the reduction of resources, shortages of staff and internal and external politics.

Seedhouse (1988) makes no distinction between ethics and morality. He states all variations of the words can be used interchangeably. In the complex world of ethics midwifery managers and midwives would be well advised to follow this advice. Not only will this assist understanding, but will help midwives deal with the tensions that accompany 'everyday ethics'. This is a term Seedhouse uses to show the difference between the intuitive reactions to life-situations and dilemmas as compared to those grounded in more abstract theory and principles.

Understanding ethics

Autonomy

Basically this is freedom of a person to decide what they will or will not do with their life, their body and their self. Personal autonomy refers to a person's capacity and ability to choose freely for herself or himself, and to be able to direct their own life. Autonomy is hardly ever absolute because it is restricted and controlled by others, through law, and health and social policy - National Health Service rationing and medical paternalism. Respect for autonomy in health care involves informed consent, which is the freedom of patients and clients to act upon the information given to them. If any element of coercion enters the situation, freedom of choice cannot be exercised.

Beneficence

The thinking behind beneficence is 'we actually have a duty to do good and prevent harm'. The actual principle of beneficence makes the point that we should try in practice to do good and not evil, and not by merely showing we wish to do so. To apply the principle of beneficence a person has to be clear what is considered as good and what is considered as evil. Midwives and doctors practice to 'do no harm', but they also act in such a way that mothers and babies will benefit from their care. To do nothing when it is required is contrary to the principle of beneficence.

Confidentiality

Patients and clients of health care expect confidentiality. In some way this is an 'unwritten contract', which allows people to give information about themselves to health professionals, information that otherwise would not be revealed. Every health professional has a duty to keep confidential any information about their patients or clients. For midwives, the following extract from the UKCC Code of Professional Conduct (1992) makes their position on confidentiality clear:

> 'As a registered nurse, midwife or health visitor, you are personally accountable for your practice, and, in the exercise of your professional accountability, must protect all confidential information concerning patients and clients obtained in the course of professional practice and make disclosures only with consent, where required by the order of a court or where you can justify disclosure in the wider public interest.'

Deontology

Deontological theories, in contrast to utilitarianism, hold that some features of acts, other than their consequences, make them right or wrong. Different deontological theories compete with each other, as well as against utilitarianism. Deontologists try in different ways to defend their judgements. That certain acts are right or wrong according to religious traditions, human reasons, law, rights, intuition and common sense. Seedhouse (1988) maintains that central to deontology is the idea that to be moral a person must perform their preordained duty, and that 'in it's purest form deontology holds that a person should always, without exception, perform certain duties whatever the consequences'. There is not one principle or duty on which all deontologists will agree.

Equality

The requirement to respect persons equally, follows from the requirement to effect autonomy in all people. People who work for the National Health Service are valuable not only because of their skills but because of 'what each person is'. Equality supports the principle that basic aspects of life are shared equally by all persons, such as being able to value one's life and having the potential for future choices. The extent people are granted equal respect is conditional on individual judgement. If mothers are not treated equally in their informed choices as to the type and place of confinement they want, and are overridden by the choices of health professionals, then according to Seedhouse (1988) this is discrimination between beings who are fundamentally equal.

Normative ethics

'General normative ethics' is an area of inquiry which seeks to answer whether actions are justly acceptable and why. Beauchamp and Childress (1989) have summarized this as an attempt to answer which 'action-guides are worthy of moral acceptance and for what reasons?'. It involves attempting to justify actions by applying them to ethical theories, which usually have a set of ethical action-guides that fulfil a number of tests. However, even if an ethical theory was totally available numerous question would remain unanswered.

'Applied normative ethics' are attempts to apply these action-guides to different moral problems. According to Beauchamp and Childress (1989) the term 'applied' refers to the use of ethical theory and methods of analysis to examine moral problems in the professions. Consequently, action-guides developed to deal with moral problems in professional practice will be shaped by moral principles, rules, models of behaviour and reflective analysis.

Nonnormative ethics

These include 'descriptive ethics' and 'metaethics' both of which can be grouped together because they do not attempt to supply prescriptive guidelines. Their objective is to establish the facts or concepts, and not the ethics in a situation. 'Descriptive ethics' is a factual inquiry of morals and beliefs. It does not examine what people ought to do but how they reason and behave. 'Methaethics' embodies the analysis of thought, concepts and language. It examines the meanings of important ethical terms, such as obligations, responsibilities and rights, and studies the logic and rationalism of moral reasoning and justification.

Utilitarianism

This moral theory considers there is only one basic principle in ethics - the principle of utility, which asserts 'that we ought always to produce the greatest possible balance of value over disvalue' (Beauchamp and Childress, 1989). In popular terms it is expressed as the theory that 'promotes the greatest good of the greatest number' and where 'the end justifies the means'. According to McNaughton (1988) in broad terms it tells us our moral duty is to 'produce as much happiness as possible'. In other words an action is justified if it produces more good than any alternative. Utilitarians believe that telling lies, manipulation, deceit and other actions that are traditionally considered to be morally wrong are 'morally neutral' when they lead to the best consequences. Beauchamp and Childress (1989) assert all utilitarians 'share the conviction that human actions are to be morally assessed in terms of their production of maximal nonmoral value'. In reality, some utilitarians believe pursuance of the best circumstances is the only factor, while others consider one view should be balanced against those of another.

Veracity

In health care truth-telling has been debated for a long time, but in recent years there is a growing consensus that the patient has a right to know the truth. Truthfulness is central to the principle of conduct. The professional's responsibility to give full information is not in dispute, but are there instances when to give full information will cause harm? Is to withhold information lying? Today, respect for autonomy involves a patient having the right to receive or not to receive information.

Information technology and computers are progressively being used to store information about patients and their personal records. Under European law everyone has a right to examine computer data held on them, and in consequence some British patients are now gaining access and reading their own medical files. Now that mothers carry their own pregnancy health records, this has removed the mystique of the 'old style of obstetric case notes'. By encouraging mothers to keep their notes, and to share and read what has been written and recorded, there should be little room for misinterpretation and misunderstanding.

Codes of professional ethics

The UKCC Code of Professional Conduct (1992) and the Midwife's Code of Practice (1994) provide specific rules for practice and professional accountability. However, it is important that midwives know the difference between professional codes and general moral codes. Beauchamp and Childress (1989) assert 'professional codes specify action-guides for a particular group which are justified by reference to general principles and rules', but general moral codes consist of 'society's cherished moral principles and rules' e.g. people who promise to do something have a moral obligation to do it.

Codes of professional conduct are an attempt to classify and enforce primary responsibilities and obligations, so that professionals are competent and trustworthy when involved with people they 'care for' or come into contact with. However, as Salvage (1984) observed ethical codes are not 'tablets of stone engraved with a list of prohibitions'. When professional codes contain defensible moral principles they are effective but when oversimplified could be ineffective. The problem with oversimplification is that professionals may believe they have satisfied the moral requirements by solely following the rules of the code, and not applying normative ethics. The examination of real situations when ethical problems arise will usually involve a conflict of values. Generally there are more questions than answers. Salvage (1984) believes this is how it should be. Professionals cannot look for concrete answers, but must consider carefully how they go about making decisions each day, and recognizing the ethical dimension of their roles. Clarke (1995) asserts that the values contained in the UKCC professional codes are 'consistent with the values that a caring profession should promote'. However, she believes the daily practice of midwives demonstrates behaviour, decision-making and attitudes which 'still lean towards fulfilling the utilitarian goals of the NHS' and not the individual needs of women. For professional codes to be effectual they need to include veracity, respect for autonomy and justice, and not only the principles of beneficence and confidentiality which is frequently the case.

Accountability

The word 'accountable' originates from the metaphor of 'keeping account' of one's conduct (Buttny, 1993). To be accountable to others arises from the condition that persons can be held responsible for their actions. In almost all social situations the necessity for 'accounts' will emerge. These can range from offering an excuse for arriving late to defending one's actions when accused of misconduct. Accounts can be recognized in everyday language as apologies, excuses, explanations, justifications, descriptions and defences. Actions can be said to be done correctly or carelessly, successfully or ineffectively, or competently or incompetently. As a consequence a person will warrant varying degrees of praise or blame. According to Buttny (1993) 'blame, and critical judgements underpinning it, reflect our ontological condition as moral beings'. The human capacity to be blamed and held responsible for one's actions is what creates the necessity for 'accounts' and accountability.

Being held accountable for failure reflects certain assumptions about human action and performance. For example, a midwife seen to be competent who yet makes errors in performance may be held accountable. Repeated errors will lead to questions about the midwife's competence. The most serious type of failure involves 'improper intentions'. Intentions, such as 'effort' are considered to be more controllable than 'ability'. Therefore, a midwife will be held responsible for what she can control. Thus it can be seen that failures due to 'lack of ability' reflect a midwife's competence, whilst failures due to 'improper intentions' reflect a midwife's moral character. The notion that nurses and midwives should be accountable for their practice, to themselves, to patients and clients and to each other, 'contains with it certain ethical assumptions or value judgements' (Salvage, 1984). The UKCC advisory document *Exercising Accountability* (1989) provides a valuable framework for nurses, midwives and health visitors when considering ethical aspects of their professional practice and exercising accountability.

However, the notion of 'constraints' can also implicate a limitation in a midwife's abilities. This follows that midwives should only be held accountable for those activities and outcomes which they can exercise and control. Buttny (1993) believes that 'inevitability' limits responsibility. Only by having a 'realm of inevitability' can areas over which one has no control be defined. The realm of inevitability is usually associated with bodily functions and its limitations. For example, a midwife who is tired and unable to concentrate due to being on call and working most of the night has an excusing condition for not reporting on duty. Constraints associated with excessive workload, shortages of staff and lack of resources could all limit a midwife's ability to practice safely. In these circumstances where does the responsibility lie? Midwives are advised to inform their midwifery manager when a potentially 'constraining' situation arises, but whose responsibility does it become then? Is it still the midwife or does responsibility pass to the midwifery manager? Where does accountability lie when situations cannot always be resolved? By reporting such situations does not mean midwives can absolve all accountability, but by sharing the problem at least midwives and managers have the opportunity to do something to resolve the situation.

Verbal and written accounts as a 're-presentation' of actions and events can be fraught with difficulties. Yet they form an essential part of accountability. For example, a number of staff may observe a person physically attack another, but what exactly did they see? The social and moral significance of the event cannot be sufficiently recapitulated by simply describing physical actions. To know what really happened, their needs to be information about the perpetrators intention, related history, background knowledge and circumstances. A 're-presentation' combined with shared knowledge and cultural assumptions can transform the significance of the event. The same could apply when a midwife has to provide a 're-presentation account' of an event she was involved in e.g. concerning her professional practice, or during a complaint investigation. Generally recipients of accounts, midwifery managers, supervisors of midwives, attend to both the representational and presentational functions. However, Buttny (1993) believes that recipients are often 'less interested in the account's veracity and more concerned with maintaining the ongoing interaction and relationship', and thus the resolution is more through negotiation and seeking alignment.

Business ethics

Business ethics are an applied discipline, which McHugh (1991) asserts may be fascinating but not useful if people in business are not helped to make moral decisions. He says making ethical decisions is not easy. Research and hard work are required in order to clarify and describe real situations, so as to be able to set down rules and values.

NHS Trusts

The directors of NHS Trusts, both executive and non-executive, have moral responsibilities to:

- managers
- employees
- customers
- suppliers
- the local community
- the NHS Management Executive Board.

Dilemmas can arise for directors as with all health service workers in trying to satisfy the full range of their responsibilities. These include company policy, resource allocation, efficient use of resources and meeting the conditions and standards as agreed in contracts with purchasers. The need for efficiency and effectiveness is a tension, but directors have a duty to keep the thrust of business in balance with providing a health service which meets the needs of the local population. Financial success is important, but it is not the only measure. Business ethics takes account of the values and practices in the organization, and are a reminder that the NHS Trust exists to serve the people. By developing a corporate culture, which is open and involves staff in objectives and goals, and setting a mutually agreed business strategy, everyone in the NHS Trust should be committed to providing high quality health care.

In some respects, although NHS Trusts are not persons, the ideas and functions that are applied to a person can be applied to a Trust e.g. goals, values, plans etc. McHugh refers to this as the 'Company Conscience'. The 'effective voice of conscience' he says, lies in the leadership of directors and managers who provide that crucial link between individual and organizational values. Consumer pressure and public opinion can also influence the company conscience.

Ethics and employment

Employment is a dynamic changing situation. It is one in which midwifery managers representing employers, and staff, and the employees, respond to one another. Due to uncertain conditions of the NHS internal market this may affect contracts and finance and may result in changes having to be made in employment practices and working conditions. Employment should be one of 'partnership', in which a recognition in the needs of the managers and staff can flow freely between each other and be responsive. Unfortunately this is not always the case.

The midwifery manager, in her role of appointing midwives has an ethical duty to ensure they are competent in their practice, are contented, have job satisfaction and enjoy their work. This ethical duty is based on the belief that staff who are dissatisfied and unhappy do not perform so effectively, and therefore put mothers and babies at risk.

Midwives, on the other hand, when in employment will receive a salary, will gain skills and experience in their work, will gain additional knowledge through continuing and in-service education, and will benefit through the wider socialization with others.

In brief, both employers and employees have duties as follows:

*   duties of employers:
    - to encompass active ethical and moral principles
    - accountability for the welfare of staff e.g. health and safety and fairness.

*   duties of employees
    - not to carry out wrong practices, or do anything unethical in the course of their work e.g. malpractice and misconduct.

The ethical responsibilities for midwifery managers are many and varied. These include the appointment of new staff and the promotion of selected staff to more senior positions. Not only is it important to ensure a person is right for the job, but it is essential the person appointed will fit into the culture of the organization. Each of the following responsibilities have numerous ethical dimensions, and need to be examined carefully to guarantee that a person is treated fairly and with respect (also see Chapter 5 - Managing Resources).

Recruitment

- how is the advert worded?
- internal or external advertising?
- is the 'person specification' for the job clear?
- equal opportunities?

Short-listing

- how objective is it?
- does it involve those who will be on the interview panel?

Interview

- the conduct of the interview
- the venue, the room layout and accessibility
- the number on the interview panel
- the standard of questions; is there two way communication?
- have any special tests been used?
- how objective is the final selection?
- references - written or verbal; what is said or not said
- health questionnaire and medical clearance.

Post-interview

- Is counselling offered?
- telephone or face to face counselling?
- honesty and openness.

Appointment

OFFER
- by telephone or letter?
- registration check with UKCC.

ACCEPTANCE
- induction or orientation programme and evaluation.

Continuing employment

- does the employee expect no change in contract hours?
- are individual performance reviews carried out?

- is good work and effort rewarded?
- how is failure to maintain standards handled?
- how is sickness and absenteeism monitored?
- are grievance and disciplinary issues dealt with fairly?

Retirement
- preparation for planned retirement and is there celebration?
- reasons for early retirement
- reasons for redundancy.

Ethical and moral leadership

Ethical leadership is about taking responsibility for one's commitments and one's choices. Midwifery managers and midwifery sisters in choosing and accepting their combined management and professional roles, take on responsibilities that go with the job. In doing so they will find themselves involved in ethical dilemmas, not only those perceived by themselves, but those perceived by other midwives and other health professionals. It follows then, that they will be expected to take a lead and provide guidance on how to deal with some of these dilemmas.

What style of leadership to use in these situations is an interesting one. Wall (1989) argues that the style the manager chooses has ethical significance. He assumes leading from the front implies leaders know where they are going, leading from the middle is 'uncharismatic' and leading from behind suggests some sort of manipulation. The point of looking at these simple images of leadership, he suggests, is that the manager has to feel right about their style of leadership (see Chapter 2). He concludes all managers need to explore their leadership style to ensure that their practice of management is not only effective, but also, 'in an ethical sense, good'.

Providing leadership

In attempting to provide leadership in the management of ethical dilemmas, there are several things midwifery managers and midwifery sisters can do:

- create an open culture - one in which the staff have respect for each other and feel confident in their own practice and the practice of others
- know about ethics - have a basic knowledge of ethical principles and the issues that can arise in everyday ethics in maternity care and midwifery practice
- issue guidelines on confidentiality - and ensure all staff sign a confidentiality clause
- issue information, guidance and discuss with staff on how to deal with:
  - untoward incidents
  - 'near misses' - where there are lesson to be learnt and shared with others to avoid something similar occurring again in the future
  - incompetence and malpractice of colleagues

- provide support through:
  - facilitating 'staff support groups'
  - providing education and training on: ethical principles, everyday ethics
  - ethical dilemmas in midwifery practice
- reflect on problems and challenges - how they occurred, why they occurred, how they were dealt with, and could they have been dealt with differently.
- discuss everyday ethics and ethical dilemmas with:
  - senior managers and the Clinical Director
  - medical and professional colleagues
  - the NHS Trust Director of Nursing and Midwifery
  - other midwives through 'networking', membership of professional organizations, study days, seminars etc.
- demonstrate through own behaviour and conduct - so there is no perceived 'gap' between what is said and what is done. Nevertheless, it is also important that staff know of the difficulty midwifery managers have to act with integrity all of the time
- apply basic human values - in decision-making and when taking actions.

The Institute of Health Services Management (1995) have produced a statement on Primary Values for managers which gives guidance when making decisions personally, as individuals and on behalf of their organization. These include:

- respect the dignity of every individual
- respect and welcome diversity among patients, colleagues and the public
- listen to the views of others
- use resources responsibly
- promote a climate in which patients, colleagues and the public can register concerns and where discussion is encouraged and valued
- take personal responsibility
- be sensitive to the consequences for others of their actions.

Some dilemmas midwifery managers may encounter

Reduction in maternity services budget

This may be as a result of external factors. For example, a reduction in the projected fertility rates for women of childbearing age or a change in purchaser contracts. Whatever the reason, this means the midwifery manager will be required to review resources, and will be under pressure to reduce the number of staff in post, particularly midwives who are considered expensive resources. The dilemma for the midwifery manager is a reduction in midwives may mean standards could fall, which would have an adverse effect on the quality of care for each mother and baby.

Health cost restrictions and scarce resources for maternity care

The amount of resources allocated to the National Health Service is finite. This is because the Department of Health has to compete with other government departments for resources each year. Scarce resources allocated at local level mean the midwifery manager may be pressed to reduce the number of midwives and appoint more maternity care assistants, at less cost. The result could be an imbalance in the Maternity Services skill-mix. A further dilemma could result if NHS Trusts' decide not to support the training of pre registration midwives but increase the training of maternity care assistants locally.

Value for money in maternity care

This is a continuing dilemma for midwifery managers. There is a responsibility to keep costs to a minimum through efficiency and effectiveness, but also a requirement to provide a high quality Maternity Services that meets the needs of every mother and baby. This requires a fine balancing act, which at times can result in the midwifery manager having to make decisions that may be misunderstood. A managerial ethic is to keep within budget and the finances allocated, but unfortunately some midwives, clinicians and members of the public do not appreciate this, and this can create an atmosphere of misinterpretation. Efficiency is ethically correct in that it maintains the principle of maximizing benefit.

Helping midwives to deal with moral situations

In providing care midwives frequently find themselves asking 'what is the morally right thing for me to do?'. This involves making judgements observed from several viewpoints including law, professional codes, social 'norms', religious beliefs, political objectives and practical outcomes. The difficulty with making a judgement is that midwives may see moral judgements as different from legal and religious ones, and their feelings may disagree with the views of mothers and colleagues. In these situations midwives have to 'delve deeper' to try to answer more questions, such as:

- is it important to follow certain feelings more than others, and why?
- can any reasons be found, which are acceptable to mothers, self and colleagues, for acting one way rather than another?
- is there a compromise which may be morally acceptable?

According to Rowson (1992), there are four main moral positions which midwives can use to understand their own and other people's perspective and to help identify sources of disagreement when there are different views as to what should be done:

1. To act morally we must try to produce the best consequences. As there is a moral obligation to bring about the best outcome, alternative actions and their effect on others must be considered before deciding which action will bring about the greatest benefit and the least harm. The basic view is that 'the end justifies the means' - in other words it involves using 'whatever means to achieve the best circumstances'. Telling lies, deceit and breaking promises are accepted as long as it leads to the best consequence. This view is 'utilitarianism' or 'consequentialism' and works on the principle that actions are valuable only if useful and lead to the best consequences.

2. To act morally we must carry out actions which are right in themselves and avoid actions which are wrong. Some people will find the 'utilitarian' view

unacceptable. They consider telling lies, deception, betraying trust are wrong in themselves, and it is their moral duty to avoid them. Likewise they believe always telling a person the truth whether or not it is in 'their best interests' and they never take actions which are wrong in themselves. This is known as the 'dutiful view'. The motivation is to do the right action because it is right and not because of any likely benefit that will result.

3. To act morally we must treat people justly and fairly. Generally people believe others should be valued equally and treated alike, unless there is a difference between them which will necessitate treating them differently. People are regarded as equally important regardless of their race, nationality, gender, religion, age etc. However, differences in medical conditions would justify giving different treatments to those who present with different symptoms. This view is known as the principle of 'justice' or 'fairness'. People and their interests should be valued equally, and if anyone wants to treat them differently they must show the differences that are relevant to treatment.

4. To act morally we must respect autonomy for others. People should respect other people's freedom to make their own decisions. When people have the ability to understand and assess their own situation they can make informed choices. Consequently it is morally wrong to manipulate people. On the contrary they should be facilitated to make up their own mind, by being truthful with them. In maternity care mothers should be fully informed about their condition, alternative treatments available and their probable effects. Treatments should only continue when mothers have given their 'informed consent'. In this situation midwives would have moral obligation to accept and act in accordance with the mother's decision, rather than what they consider is in her best interests. In such situations the 'autonomy' view disagrees with 'utilitarianism'.

Some examples of dilemmas midwives may encounter:

*   a mother with a poor obstetric history wants a home confinement. She is high risk to complications during labour. Her GP has refused to be involved in her care, and intends to ask the mother to find another GP for herself and her family.

*   a mother in a 'travelling community' wants a home confinement. She lives in a caravan in a 'clearing', at least half a mile from the road. There are no main services on site, and midwives would have to walk across fields to attend her.

*   during pregnancy a mother requests the midwife not to monitor her fetus during labour, or to perform any active resuscitation measures after the baby's birth. She explains that she and her husband believe in 'non-intervention for the baby' and are prepared to take full responsibility for their decision by signing a statement which can be entered in her notes.

*   a mother refuses to let the midwife monitor the fetal heart of her second twin. The first twin was born by forceps, and there is some concern for the second twin. The midwife is pushed away as she attempts to listen to the fetal heart.

- a mother decides she wants to go home, because of personal problems, two hours following a complicated labour. She and the baby still require careful monitoring for at least another twenty four hours. She is determined to go, and says she knows the consequences of her actions.

- a baby born at 29 weeks who required maximum ventilatory support for six weeks, has developed extensive cystic changes diagnosed by cranial ultrasound. His prognosis is poor with a ninety five per cent chance of severe disability. His parents have been asked to consider whether extraordinary measures should be continued to keep him alive.

- midwives in a busy postnatal ward are under considerable pressure to meet the demands of all the mothers and babies in their care. The situation has been made worse due to staff sickness. Decisions about dividing and rationing their time and attention fairly to individual mothers and babies are required.

- a midwife calls to visit a mother and baby five days after delivery. The home-visit had previously been arranged but on arrival the midwife is told the mother is not there. Her twelve year old daughter tells the midwife her mother has gone to work.

- a group of midwives have been invited to a concert and a meal afterwards, to be paid for by a representative of a 'baby milk' manufacturer. The company also markets milk in Third World countries.

Managers ethical checklist

Wall (1995) has put together a useful 'Manager's checklist' in which he identifies some of the fundamental questions managers need to consider. He states clearly that ethics cannot be bought, but are a synthesis of what the manager believes in and how they match the obligations of their job. As some aspects of this 'Manager's checklist' will be of particular value to midwifery managers, extracts are reproduced below with a few word changes e.g. 'patient' replaced by 'mother', to make it more suitable for Maternity Services use.

'Being ethical does not mean that you have to be consistent at all times, but it does require you use your judgement. The ability to do so comes from reflecting on your personal beliefs and experience'.

To this end it is useful to be able to demonstrate that you have considered the following:

- Does your organization have a statement of values? If so, have you recently asked a sample of staff if they could tell you what it says?

- Who sits on the ethical committee? Apart from junior doctor's protocols, what else does it discuss? Does it discuss, for instance, the range of services to be purchased or when to withhold treatment?

- How does the organization make choices about resources? Have you used:
  - value for money exercises
  - clinical and managerial audit
  - consumer surveys.

  How far have the results been shared with others both within and outside the organization?

- Could you give examples when you have led from the front and when you led from within the group? How did you decide what was most appropriate?

- What are your relations with voluntary bodies? What guidance is given to ensure that inappropriate work is not undertaken or that confidentiality of mothers is not breached?

- What examples can you give to demonstrate that your organization values individuals? For instance does it:
  - adapt to mothers and babies individual needs
  - respect mothers wishes
  - avoid implementing rules blindly?

- What example can you give that your organization has due regard for the interests of the communities it serves? For instance:
  - has open meetings
  - provides regular information
  - develops good press relations
  - involves the public in key decisions?

- Finally, if someone asked you how you apply ethics to your job, how would you answer?

Summary

A special type of moral leadership is required for managing the Maternity Services, which abounds with value-laden situations and where sound ethical decisions have to be made. Midwifery managers work at the centre of a work environment where tensions accompany clinical action but they must not lose sight of their management responsibilities. Midwifery managers have responsibilities to many groups of people, and it is not possible to please them all, which can cause conflict.

Ethics and morals are standards and principles of conduct which govern our behaviour and by which people judge one another. Professional practitioners and midwifery managers require knowledge and understanding of the special principles that govern maternity care. These include respect for autonomy, beneficence, confidentiality, equality and veracity. Codes of professional practice classify and enforce primary responsibilities in an attempt to ensure professionals are competent and trustworthy. Accountability arises from professionals being responsible for their actions. Verbal and written 'accounts' form an essential part of accountability.

Business ethics are required by directors of NHS Trusts, and take into account the values and principles of providing health services that meet the needs of customers. Dilemmas can arise when directors try to satisfy their full range of responsibilities, including resource allocation and balancing the annual accounts. Ethics in employment requires midwifery managers to guarantee their recruitment and selection procedures are fair, and that midwives are competent to practice and have job satisfaction. Midwives in return have a duty not to do anything unethical or to carry out wrong practice in the course of their work.

Ethical dilemmas in midwifery practice and management do not happen daily but midwifery managers must be able to recognize, define, discuss and examine ethical situations with professional and obstetric colleagues, using known principles of ethics. This will help midwives with their judgements and to deal with moral situations more successfully. Judgements can be perceived from several viewpoints and midwives may find their feelings disagree with the views of mothers and colleagues. Dilemmas for midwifery managers are usually associated with the restriction of resources and keeping costs to a minimal.

Wall (1995) has produced a 'Managers Ethical Checklist' which will help midwifery managers identify some of the fundamental questions they need to consider as they go about their daily work.

References

Adair, J. (1986). *Effective Teambuilding.* London: Gower Publishing Company Ltd.

Andrews, A. (1994). 'Managing your manager'. *Nursing Standard*, April, Vol. 8, No. 31, pp.49-54.

Argyle, M. (1979). *The Social Psychology of Work.* Harmondsworth, Middlesex: Penguin Books Ltd.

Association of Radical Midwives (1986). *The Vision. Proposals for the Future of Maternity Services.* Ormskirk: ARM.

Atwood, M. (1985). *Introduction to Personal Management.* London: Pan Books Ltd.

Auld, M.G. (1992). 'Quality who says what?'. *Midwives Chronicle & Nursing Notes.* December, Vol. 105, No. 1259, pp.378-385.

Barnett, E. (1989). 'Midwives take on their critics'. *Daily News.* November, p.10.

Baron, L. (1979). 'Home or hospital delivery?'. *Midwife Health Visitor and Community Nurse.* March, Vol. 15, No. 3, pp.94-95.

Beauchamp, T.L., Childress, J.F. (1989). *Principles of Biomedical Ethics.* Oxford: Oxford University Press.

Beekman, D. (1979). *The Mechanical Baby.* London: Dennis Dobson.

Belbin, R., Meredith (1991). *Management Teams - Why They Succeed or Fail.* Oxford: Butterworth-Heinemann Ltd.

Benton, D. (1994). 'Management and leadership'. *Nursing Standard*, April. Vol 8, No 29, pp.49-54.

Betty, I. (1995). 'The driving force'. *The Health Service Journal.* Vol.105, No. 5447, April. p.31.

Blake, J., Lawrence, P. (1989). *The ABC of Management.* London: Casell Educational.

Bond, M., Holland, S. (1988). 'Stress and tension control'. *Beating Aggression.* pp.13-45. London: Weidenfeld and Nicholson Ltd.

Boot, R.L., Cowling, A.G., Stanworth, M.J.K. (1982). *Behavioural Sciences.* London: Edward Arnold (Publishing) Ltd.

Buckley, K.W., Steffy, J. (1986). 'The invisible side of leadership'. *Transforming Leadership.* pp.233-243. Virginia, USA: Miles River Press.

Business Now (1994). *How to Respond When They're Piling on the Pressure.* Issue 21, July. Wyvern Crest Ltd.

Buttny, R. (1993). *Social Accountability in Communication.* London: Sage.

Cava, R. (1991). *Dealing with Difficult People.* London: Piatkus (Publishers) Ltd.

Clarke, R.A. (1995). 'Ethics and midwifery practice' *Midwives.* August, Vol.108, No. 1291, pp.270-271.

Cooper, D.B. (1994). 'The standard guide to communication'. *Nursing Standard.* April, Vol. 8, No. 29, pp.42-43.

Cowell, B., Wainright, D. (1981). *Behind the Blue Door.* London: Balliere Tindall.

Cross, R.E., Craven, R., Hudson, M., Reynolds, V. (1991). *Midwifery Care in Practice.* West Midlands Region - Heads of Midwifery Services.

Da Cruz, V. (1967). *Mayes' Handbook of Midwifery.* Seventh Edition. London: Bailliere, Tindall and Cassell.

Davidson, M. (1985). *Reach for the Top.* London: Judy Piatkus (Publishers) Ltd.

Davies, P. (1991). 'News focus - IPR is put through its paces and found wanting'. *The Health Service Journal.* 19th September.

Deighan, M. (1993). 'Is anybody out there listening?' *Nursing Standard.* September, Vol 8, No 1, p.9.

Department of Health (1989). *Working for Patients.* London: HMSO.

Department of Health (1991). *The Patient's Charter.* London: HMSO

Department of Health (1992). *Maternity Services, Government Response to the Second Report from the Health Committee Session 91-92.* London: HMSO.

Department of Health (1993). *Changing Childbirth: The Report of the Expert Maternity Group.* London: HMSO.

Department of Health (1994). *The Challenge for Nursing and Midwifery In the 21st Century.* London: HMSO.

Department of Health (1995). *NHS The Patients Charter Maternity Services.* London: London: HMSO.

Dixon, P., Carr-Hill, R. (1989). 'Customer feedback surveys - An introduction to survey methods'. *The NHS and its Customers.* University of York: Centre for Health Economics.

Donnison, J. (1988). *Midwives and Medical Men.* London: Historical Publications Ltd.

Drummond, H. (1991). *Power: Creating it Using it.* London: Kogan Page Ltd.

Drummond, H. (1991). *Effective Decision Making.* London: Kogan Page Ltd.

Eggert, M. (1994). 'Team playing', *Nursing Standard.* April. Vol. 8, No. 28, pp.49-56.

Fanning, M. (1994). 'Don't play the blame game'. *Nursing Standard,* February. Vol 8, No 21, pp.50-51.

Fardell, J. (1994). 'Teaching and learning in practice - quality in learning'. *Nursing Times.* April, Vol. 90, No.14, pp. i-viii.

Flanagan, H. (1993). 'Managing the human resources of the NHS in the 1990s'. *The New Face of the NHS.* pp.119-145. Harlow, Essex: Longman Group UK Ltd.

Flint, C., Poulengeris, P. (1986). *The 'Know Your Midwife' Report.* London. Supported by South West Thames RHA and the Wellington Foundation.

Francis, D., Woodcock, M. (1982). 'Getting appraisal right' *Fifty Activities for Self Development.* Aldershot: Gower.

Grimley, I. (1995). 'Dilemmas of care'. *Nursing Times.* May, Vol 91, No 18 pp.42-43.

Gunning, R. (1968). *The Technique of Clear Writing.* London: McGraw Hill.

Hadridge, P. (1995). 'Tomorrow's world'. *Health Service Journal.* January, Vol. 105, No. 5447, pp.18-20.

Ham, C. (1991). *The New National Health Service.* Oxford: Radcliffe Medical Press Ltd.

Ham, C. (1993). *Health Policy in Britain.* London: The Macmillan Press Ltd.

Handy, C. (1993). *Understanding Organizations.* London: Penguin Books Ltd.

Handy, C. (1995). *Gods of Management.* London: Arrow Books Ltd.

Harding, H. (1988). *Management Appreciation.* London: Pitman Publishing.

Hickman, M. A. (1978). *An Introduction to Midwifery.* London: Blackwell Scientific Publications.

Hiley, J., Edis, M. (1992). 'Teamwork: managing a team'. *Nursing Times.* May, Vol. 88, No. 19, pp.i-viii.

Hill, J., Taylor, A. (1977). 'Fetal monitoring - a consumer viewpoint'. *The Journal of Maternal and Child Health.* December, pp.472-474.

House of Commons (1991-1992). *Health Committee, Second Report, Maternity Services.* Chairman: Winterton, N. London: HMSO.

Howe, R. J., Gaeddert, D., Howe, M.A. (1993). *Quality on Trial.* Maidenhead, Berkshire: McGraw - Hill Book Company Europe.

Hunt, J. (1983). *Managing People at Work.* London: Pan Books Ltd.

Jackson, K. (1995). 'Changing Childbirth: Encouraging debate' *British Journal of Midwifery.* March, Vol. 3, No. 3, pp.137-138.

Jacquerye, A. (1994). 'The cost of quality' - supplement euroquan'. *Nursing Standard.* March, Vol. 8, No. 24.

Jordan, M. (1987). 'Just right for the job'. *Nursing Times.* October, Vol. 83, No. 42, pp.45-46.

Kelsall, B. (1993). 'Are midwives ready for consumer-led care' *Professional Care of Mother and Child.* February. p.52.

Kelso, I., Parsons, R., Lawrence, G., Arora, S., Edmonds, D., Cooke, I. (1978). 'An assessment of continuous fetal heart rate monitoring in labour'. *American Journal of Obstetrics and Gynaecology.* July, Vol.131, No. 5, pp. 526-532.

Kinsman, F. (1986). 'Leadership from alongside'. *Transforming Leadership.* Virginia. USA: Miles River Press. pp.19-28.

Kitzinger, S. (1988). *The Midwife Challenge.* London: Pandora Press.

Koch, H. (1993). 'Buying and selling high-quality health care'. *The New Face of the NHS.* pp.146-159. Harlow, Essex: Longman Group UK Limited.

La Monica, E. L. (1994). *Management in Health Care (British Adaptation).* London: Macmillan Press Ltd.

Lamplugh, D. (1988). *Beating Aggression.* London: Wiedenfeld & Nicholson Ltd.

Lee-Potter, L. (1995). 'A baby taken seriously'. *Daily Mail.* June 14. p.9.

Maddux, R.B. (1989). *Effective Performance Appraisals.* London: Kogan Page Ltd.

Magill-Cuerden, J. (1992). 'A question of communication'. *Modern Midwife.* November/December, Vol. 2, No. 6, pp.4-5.

Maloney, E.M. (1994). 'Managerial ethics'. *Management in Health Care.* pp. 118-133. London: The Macmillan Press Ltd.

Mangan, P. (1994). 'Strategies for success'. *Nursing Times,* April, Vol. 90, No. 14.

Mathieson, A., Kellet, J. (1994). 'Personal power'. *Nursing Standard.* March 30. Vol. 8, No. 27.

Mauksch, I.G., Miller, M.H. (1981). *Implementing Change in Nursing.* St Louis: CV Mosby.

McCormack, M. H. (1985). *What They Don't Teach You At Harvard Business School.* London: Guild Publishing.

McHugh, F.P. (1991). *Ethics in Business Now.* London: Macmillan Education Ltd.

McIver, S., Carr-Hill, R. (1989). 'A survey of the current practice of customer relations'. *The NHS and its Customers.* University of York: Centre for Health Economics.

McNaughton, D. (1988). *Moral Vision.* Oxford: Basil Blackwell.

Melia, K.M. (1987). 'Everyday ethics for nursing'. *Nursing Times.* August, Vol. 83, No 31, pp.43-45.

Melia, K.M. (1989). *Everyday Nursing Ethics.* London: Macmillan Education Ltd.

Mole, P. (1993). *Acupuncture.* Dorset: Element Books.

Morgan, P. (1994). *Management in Health Care* (British Adaptation). London: Macmillan Press Ltd.

Morris, D. (1977). *Manwatching.* London: Jonathan Cape.

Munro-Faure, L., Munro-Faure, M. (1992). *Implementing Total Quality Management.* London: Pitman Publishing.

National Association of Health Authorities and Trusts (1993). *Complaints Do Matter.* Birmingham: NAHAT.

Nelson, M. J. (1992). *Managing Health Professionals.* London: Chapman & Hall.

O'Brien, M. (1981). *The Politics of Reproduction.* London: Routledge and Kegan Paul.

O'Brien, P. (1992). *Assertiveness.* London: The Industrial Society Press.

Odent, M. (1986). *Primal Health.* London: Century Hutchinson Ltd.

Overall, C. (1987). *Ethics and Human Reproduction.* London: Allen and Unwin.

Overall, C. (1989). *The Future of Human Reproduction.* Toronto: The Women's Press.

PA International Management Consultants Ltd. (1975). *Report Writing.* Kent: Multimedia Take-Away Guide.

Pearson, B., Thomas, N. (1991). *The Shorter MBA - A Practical Approach to Business Skills.* London: Thorsons, An Imprint of Harper Collins Publishers.

Pemberton, M. (1982). *A Guide to Effective Meetings.* London: The Industrial Society Press.

Perrin, J. (1990). *Resource Management in the NHS.* London: Chapman and Hall Ltd.

Peters, T. (1990). *Thriving on Chaos.* London: Macmillan Ltd.

Piercy, J., Downe, S. (1995). 'Changing Childbirth - assessing the cost'. *Changing Childbirth Update.* June, Issue 2.

Pink, V. (1994). 'Pulling up the pill pushers' *Nursing Standard.* January, Vol 8, No 16, p.42.

Prescott, E. (1995). 'Alerting mums to be watchful'. *West Midlands Review.* April.

Read, T. (1994). 'Midwives hail push for women's choice' *Nursing Times*. February, Vol 90, No 5.

Ritscher, J. A. (1986). 'Spiritual leadership'. *Transforming Leadership*. Virginia

Robertson, D. (1993). *Violence in Your Workplace*. London: Souvenir Press (Educational and Academic) Ltd.

Robinson, S. (1989). 'Caring for childbearing women: the interrelationship between midwifery and medical responsibilities'. *Midwives, Research and Childbirth - Volume 1*. London: Chapman and Hall. pp.8-41.

Roger, D., Nash, P. (1995). 'Stress - cracking points'. *Nursing Times*. Vol.91, No. 25, June, pp.44-45.

Rogers, R., Salvage, J. (1988). *Nurses at Risk*. London: Heinemann Professional Publishing Ltd.

Rowe, D. (1992). *Wanting Everything*. London: Harper Collins Publishers.

Rowson, R. (1992). 'Ethics and care-making judgements'. *Nursing Times*. June, Vol. 88, No. 24, pp.i-viii.

Royal College of Midwives (1987). *Towards A Healthy Nation - A Policy for the Maternity Services*. London: RCM.

Royal College of Nursing (1991). *The Role of the Support Worker within the Professional Nursing Team*. London: RCN. Order No. 000150.

Salvage, J. (1984). 'Ethics - in search of answers' *Senior Nurse*. October, Vol. 1, No. 28, p.3.

Seedhouse, D. (1988). *Ethics The Heart of Health Care*. Chicester: John Wiley and Sons.

Schurr, M. (1968). *Leadership and the Nurse*. London: English Universities Press.

Scriptographic Publication. (1990). *Quality and You*. Alton, Hampshire: Scriptographic Publications Ltd.

Shine, B. (1991). *Mind Magic*. London: Bantam Press.

Shulman, A. D., Penman, R. (1981). 'Non-Verbal Communication' Contact: Human Communication and its History. London: Thames & Hudson.

Sleep, J., Grant, A., Garcia, J., Elbourne, D., Spencer, J., Chalmers, I. (1984). 'West Berkshire perineal management trial'. *British Medical Journal*. September, Vol. 289, pp.587-590.

Song, L.J. (1981). 'Quality control circles - in the civil service?' *Management Development*, July, No 32, Management Services Department and the Institute of the Singapore Civil Service.

Spurgeon, P. (1993). 'Resource management : a fundamental change in managing health services'. *The New Face of the NHS*. pp.72-85. Harlow, Essex: Longman Group UK Ltd.

Spurgeon, P. (1993). *The New Face of the NHS*. Harlow: Longman Group UK Ltd.

Stevenson, H. (1987). 'If the model fits'. *Health Service Journal*. December, p.1446.

Strong, P., Robinson, J. (1992). *The NHS - Under New Management*. Buckingham: Open University Press.

Sutherland, S. (1992). *Irrationality - The Enemy Within*. London: Constable.

Sweet, B.R. (1982). *Mayes' Midwifery*. Tenth Edition. London: Bailliere Tindall

Taylor, A. (1995). 'Absence record'. *Nursing Times*. June, Vol.91, No. 23, pp.20-21.

Taylor, N. (1992). *Budgeting Skills: A Guide for Nurse Managers*. Lancaster: Quay Publishing Ltd.

The Open University., Health Education Council., Scottish Health Education Unit. (1980). *The Good Health Guide*. London: Harper & Row Publishers.

Thompson, D. (1993). 'Developing Managers for the 1990s'. *The New Face of the NHS*. Harlow: Essex. Longman Group Uk Ltd. pp.102-118.

Thorwald, J. (1962). *Science and Secrets of Early Medicine*. London: Thames and Hudson.

Tilley, I. (1993). *Managing the Internal Market*. London: Paul Chapman Publishing Ltd.

Torrington, D., Hall, L. (1991). *Personnel Management*. Hemel Hempstead: Prentice Hall International (UK) Ltd.

Toynbee, P. (1986). 'Natural Childbirth, a child of the sixties, was and is largely a nutty fad from a noisy group of lentil-eating earth goddesses' *The Guardian*. May 12.

Treacy, D. (1991). *Clear Your Desk*. London: Century Business Books Ltd.

Tyes, S. (1982). *Communication Study Guide*. Essex: Anglian Regional Management Centre.

Tylczak, L. (1991). *Attacking Absenteeism*. London: Kogan Page Ltd.

UKCC. (1992). *Code of Professional Conduct for Nurses, Midwives and Health Visitors.* London: UKCC.

UKCC (1994). *The Midwife's Code of Practice.* UKCC: London.

Vaughan, B., Pillmoor, M. (1989). *Managing Nursing Work.* Harrow, Middlesex: Scutari Press.

Wall, A. (1989). *Ethics and the Health Service Manager.* London: Kings Fund Publishing.

Wall, A., Cole, A. (1995). 'Ethics and probity'. *Health Management Guides.* May. London: Health Service Journal, Macmillan Magazines Ltd.

Walton, I., Hamilton, M. (1995). *Midwives and Changing Childbirth.* Hale, Cheshire: Books for Midwives Press.

Walton, M. (1988). *Management and Managing.* London: Harper & Row Publishers.

Walton, P. (1990). *Job Sharing - A Practical Guide.* London: Kogan Page Ltd.

Watkin, B. (1978). 'Leadership and making decisions' *Nursing Mirror Supplement.* June 22

Witz, A. (1992). *Professions and Patriarchy.* London: Routledge.

Index

Q

quality 163, 167, 174, 180
  care 165
  defining 164
  improvement 176
  meaning of 164
  objectives 174
  targets 175
quality chain 166, 169
quality circles 172
  benefits of 173
  characteristics of 172
  leader 173
quality culture 169
questionnaire distribution 179

R

rationality 47
re-presentation 188
  account 188
realm of inevitability 187
recruitment 95
  methods 96
  process 97
reduction in budget 192
references 106
refreezing 68
report writing 157
  effective 157
reporting 180
Resource Management Iniative (RMI) 86
resources 80
  categories of 80
  definition of 80
  information 67
  management 9, 79, 89
  scarce for maternity care 192
responsibility 40
restraining forces 71, 73
reward packages 95
rewards 62, 67
Ritscher (1986) 37
Robertson (1993) 133
Robinson and Strong (1992) 87
Royal College of Midwives (RCM) 8

S

safety at work 132
scientific model 55

Vroom and Yetton 51, 55
secondary resources 81
  nature of 83
  problems with 83
secretary 41
security
  measures 121
  of buildings 139
  of staff 139
selected candidate 104
selection
  methods of 99
  poor 99
selection interview 101
  briefing 102
  conducting 104
  panel 102
  plan 105
  process 105
  timing 102
  venue 103
self defence 138
self-management 41
self-motivation 39
self-respect 33
Sharpe, Jane 2
Short Report (1979-80) 15
shortlisting 98
situation theory 29
skill levels 128
skill mix 93
skills 67
  responding 152
Sleep et al (1984) 17
Smellie, William 3
social learning theory 133
staff
  appointment of 189
  selection 95
standards 163
state certified midwife 5
statistics
  monitoring 123
  publicizing 123
status 146
strategies 76
  evaluation 78
  implementing change 75
  success 39
stress 124, 129, 131
  reaction to 124
  work-induced 141